Longevity Training-Book 7-The Science of Longevity

This book is a transcription and reproduction of the training course materials from Course #7 "The Science of Longevity"

Science and medical research can tell us a lot about longevity. This includes the history of how humanity has more than doubled our average lifespan since 1900.

Long lived plants and animals also have lot of relevant information on different aspects of longevity since they are our genetic brothers.

This book consists of transcribed videos, books and chapters, presentations, and various articles all about scientific investigations into longevity.

Longevity Training-Book 7-The Science of Longevity

Longevity Training-Book 7-The Science of Longevity

Longevity Training-Book 7-The Science of Longevity

Other books by Martin K. Ettington

<u>Spiritual and Metaphysics Books:</u>
Prophecy: A History and How to Guide
God Like Powers and Abilities
Enlightenment for Newbies
Removing Illusions to Find True
    Happiness
Using the Scientific Method to Study
    the Paranormal
A Compendium of Metaphysics and
    How to Guides (Six books
    together in one volume)
Love from the Heart
The Enlightenment Experience
Learn Your Soul's Purpose
Pursuing Enlightenment
A Modern Man's Search for Truth
Use Intuition and Prophecy to Improve
    Your Life
The Handbook of Spiritual and Energy
    Healing

<u>Longevity & Immortality:</u>
Physical Immortality: A History and
    How to Guide
The Commentaries of Living Immortals
Records of Extremely Long Lived
    Persons
Enlightenment and Immortality
Longevity Improvements from Science
The 10 Principles of Personal
    Longevity
Telomeres & Longevity
The Diets and Lifestyles of the Worlds
    Oldest Peoples
The Longevity Six Books Bundle

<u>Science Fiction:</u>
Out of This Universe
Personal Freedom-Parts 1 & 2
The Psychic Soldier Series:
    Book 1-Himalayan Journey
    Book 2-A Soldier is Born
    Book 3-Fighting For Right
    Book 4-Earth Protector
The Immortality Sci Fi Bundle

<u>The God Like Powers Series:</u>
Human Invisibility
Invulnerability and Shielding
Teleportation
Psychokinesis
Our Energy Body, Auras, and
Thoughtforms

The God Like Powers Series—
    Volume 1 Compilation

<u>The Yoga Discovery Series:</u>
Yoga-An Ancient Art Form
Hatha Yoga-Helping you Live Better
Raja Yoga-Through the Ages
The Yoga Discovery Package

<u>Business & Coaching Books:</u>
Creating, Paublishing, & Marketing
    Practitioner Ebooks
Building a Successful Longevity
    Coaching Business
Why Become a Coach?
The Professional Coaching Success
Trilogy
2020-Make Money Writing and Selling
    Books
The 2020 Handbook of High Paying
    Work Without a College Degree

<u>Science, Technology, and Misc.</u>
Future Predictions By and Engineer &
    Seer
The Unusual Science & Technology
    Bundle
The Real Atlantis-In the Eye of the
    Sahara
Are Cryptozoological Animals Real or
    Imaginary?
Real Time Travel Stories From a
    Psychic Engineer
Removing Limits On Our
    Consciousness-And
    Thinking Outside the Box
33 Incredible True Survival Stories
How to Survive Anything: From the
    Wilderness to Man Made
    Disasters
All About Mars Journeys and
    Settlement
Mining the Asteroid Belt

<u>Ancient History</u>
The Real Atlantis-In the Eye of the
Sahara
Ancient & Prehistoric Civilizations
Ancient & Prehistoric Civilizations-Book
    Two
The History of Antediluvian Giants
The Antediluvian History of Earth
Ancient Underground Cities and
    Tunnels
Strange Objects Which Should Not Exist
Strange and Ancient Places in the USA
A Theory of Ancient Prehistory And
    Giant Aliens
<u>Aliens and Space</u>

Longevity Training-Book 7-The Science of Longevity

Aliens and Secret Technology
Aliens Are Already Among Us
Designing and Building Space Colonies
Humanity and the Universe
All About Moon Bases
All About Mars Journeys and Settlement

The Space and Aliens Six Books Bundle
A Theory of Ancient Prehistory and
Giant Aliens
The Space Colonies and Space
Structures Coloring Book
All About Asteroids

<u>The Longevity Training Series</u>

(A transcription of the online Multimedia Longevity Coaching Training Program)

The Personal Longevity Training Series-Book1-Long Lived Persons
The Personal Longevity Training Series-Book2-Your Soul's Purpose
The Personal Longevity Training Series-Book3-Enable Your Life Urge
The Personal Longevity Training Series-Book4-Your Spiritual Connection
The Personal Longevity Training Series-Book5-Having Love in Your Heart
The Personal Longevity Training Series-Book6-Energy Body Health
The Personal Longevity Training Series-Book7-The Science of Longevity
The Personal Longevity Training Series-Book8-Physical Body Health
The Personal Longevity Training Series-Book9-Avoiding Accidents
The Personal Longevity Training Series-Book10-Implementing These Principles

The Personal Longevity Training Series-Books One Thru Ten

These books are all available in digital and printed formats from my
website and on Amazon, Barnes & Noble, Apple ITunes, and many other sites

My Books Website is: http://mkettingtonbooks.com

Longevity Training-Book 7-The Science of Longevity

<u>Signup for our Mailing List to get the following:</u>

1) A discount coupon for 25% discount on all books on our site

2) Occasional Notices of new books available

3) Occasional Email on other offerings of ours (Monthly)

Go to this link to sign-up:

http://personal-longevity.com/mkebooks/emailsignup/

And click this link to get the FREE 102 page Ebook titled "Secrets of Many Things"

If you have any questions about this book or other subjects please contact the Author at:

mke@mkettingtonbooks.com

Longevity Training-Book 7-The Science of Longevity

Table of Contents

Introduction

Back in 2008 I became very interested in the field of Longevity and Physical Immortality. After a lot of research this led me to my first book on the subject "Physical Immortality: A History and How to Guide". This book was pretty popular and I wanted to continue learning about Longevity and what things we could do about it in our lives.

The subject continued to fascinate me to the point that I developed a Longevity Coaching program over a couple of years starting in 2011. This online training program was multimedia—consisting of videos, my writings on longevity to read, online exercises, and tests for each of ten courses. It also included a lot of additional resources for each course including extra courses on how to become a successful Longevity Coach. A student who completed the training and tests successfully would become certified as a "Longevity Coach" and authorized to teach this material to others.

I developed a set of ten principles on longevity which are as follows:

The 10 Principles of Personal Longevity are:

- The Reality of Long Lived People
- Defining Your Purpose in Life
- Enabling the Life Urge
- Your Spiritual Health
- Having Love in Your Heart
- Energy Body Health
- The Science of Longevity
- Physical Body Health
- Using your Intuition for Safety
- Implementation of these principles

What are the 10 Principles all about?

The Reality of Long Lived People

The first principle is where I provide lots of evidence of people who have lived well over the age of 120 years old to 150-180-200, and even a 256 year old man from China:

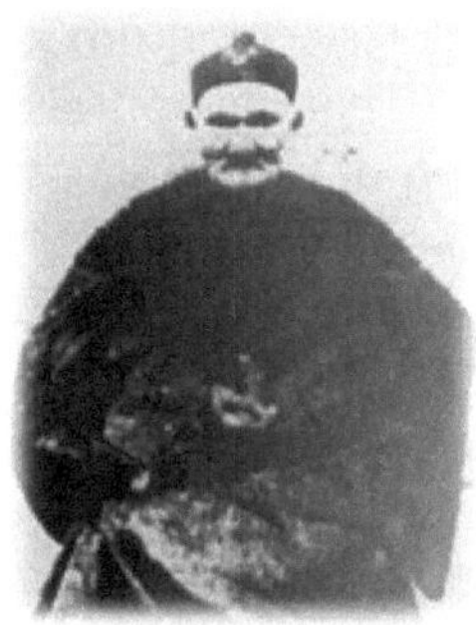

LI CHING-YUN: The Longest Lived person of record-256 Years (Source-The New York Times-May 6, 1933)

The Second Principle of Life Purpose

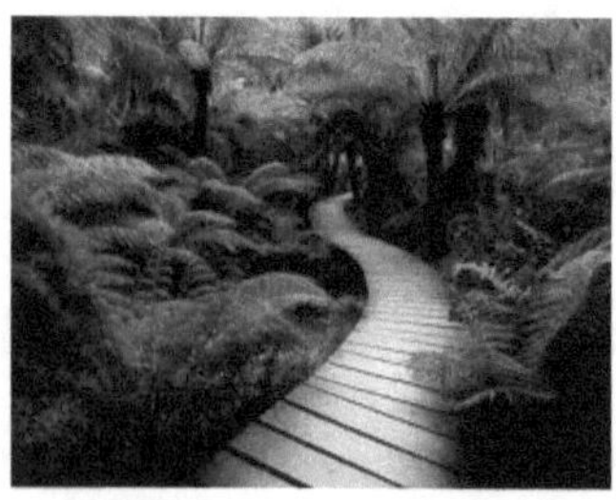

One of the things that occurred to me when I was putting the 10 principles together was that if one doesn't have a reason to live, or purpose in life--then what is the point?

This meant I had to add a very important step of how you can develop your own life purpose, or bring it up to date with your phase in life. Without reviewing your purpose-- then none of the rest of the principles matter.

Enabling the Life Urge

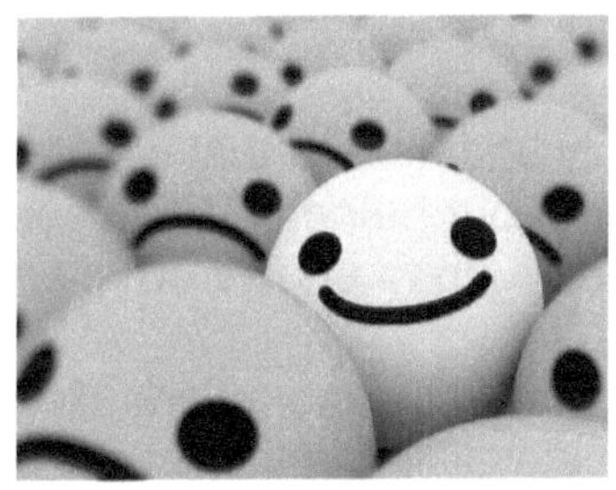

Have you ever realized how we are all programmed to expect to live through certain stages in life and then die? It's so common in our society that we don't think it odd that we expect to die at a certain age?

Have you ever heard radio ads saying "You are getting up in your sixties and seventies" so it's time to come out to our cemetery and buy a plot"

How ridiculous is this? And do you see how much our subconscious has been programmed towards death?

This principle is all about reprogramming ourselves to have a more positive outlook on life and its possibilities.

Having a Spiritual Connection in Your Life

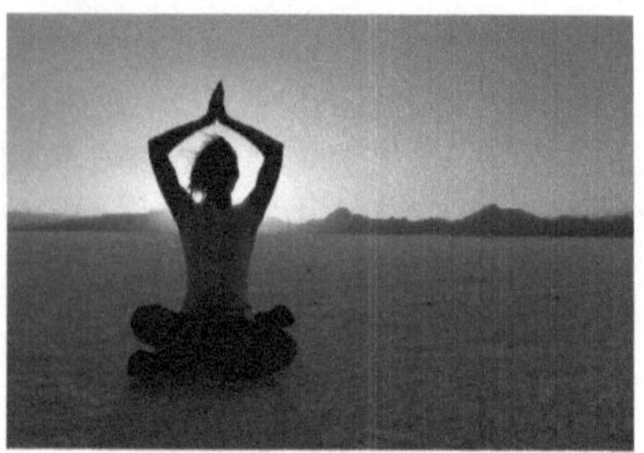

Most of us innately understand that we have a spiritual core in the center of our being. It is this spiritual core that we need to connect with to enable our physical health too.

It doesn't matter what religion you are. Regular meditation, deep prayer, or just walking in the woods helps you make and keep that connection in your life.

Having Love in Your Heart

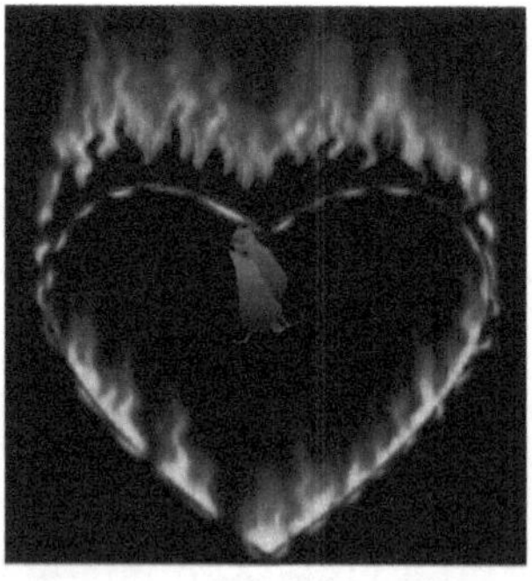

One of the most important things I learned in the last five years was that Unconditional Love is a real and physical thing. It is a powerful energy force in life and not just a philosophical belief system.

I considered it so important that I added it as a separate principle of longevity.

True Unconditional Love is healing, embodies happiness, and is a powerful part of our vital forces.

Energy Body Health

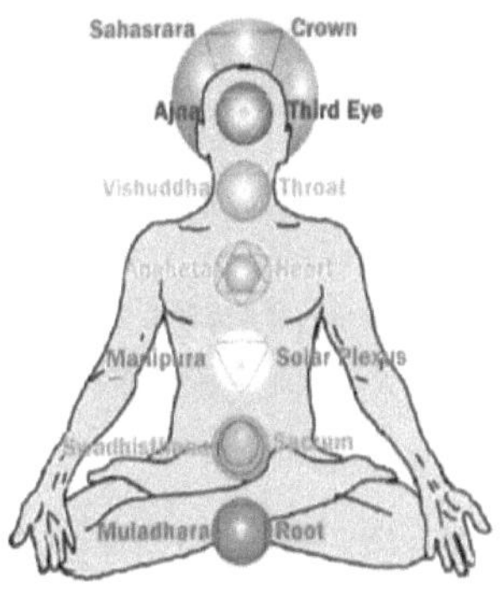

We all have an energy body which is part of our vital forces. The Indians talk about the "Chakras" and the Chinese talk about "Energy Meridians" in Acupuncture.

We should all learn different practices to keep our vital forces flowing for maximum health and vitality.

The Science of Longevity

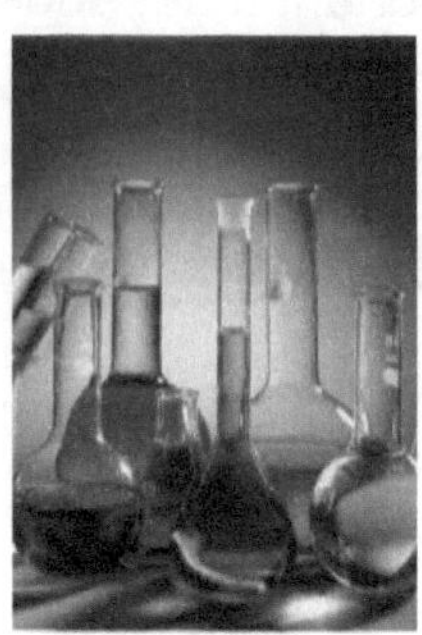

Science and Medicine are making new discoveries all the time that we can take advantage of to extend our lives. Why not take advantage of these discoveries which provide new therapies and supplements to increase our longevity.

There is also a lot we can learn from plants and animals. We all share the same genetic basis.

Some of these plants and animals live thousands of years and some cells are immortal.

What can we learn from them to apply to our lives?

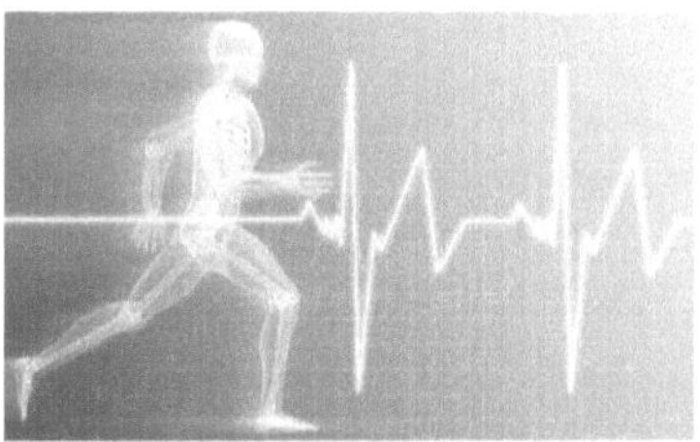

There are many types of supplements used for anti-aging for thousands of years. What can we learn about them that we can apply to our lives?

What other considerations about our physical health does nontraditional or alternative medicine offer?

Using Your Intuition for Safety

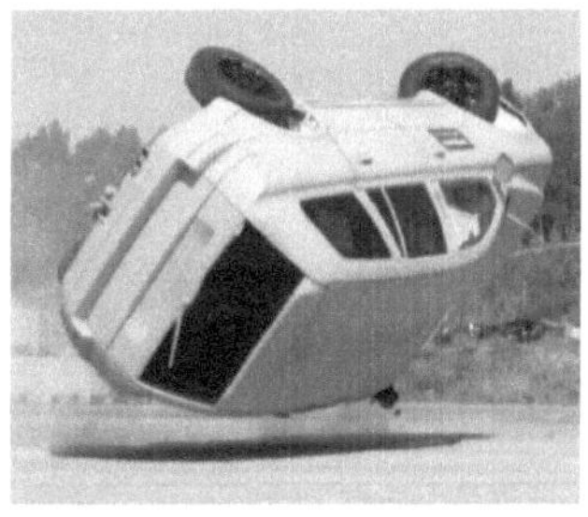

Once you have established your own long term health then what is the greatest danger you face?

ACCIDENTS

We can learn to use our intuition to make us safer as well as see potential future events which may be good too.

Why not open up to the possibilities of how our spirit has this natural ability in all of us?

Implementing These Principles in Your Life

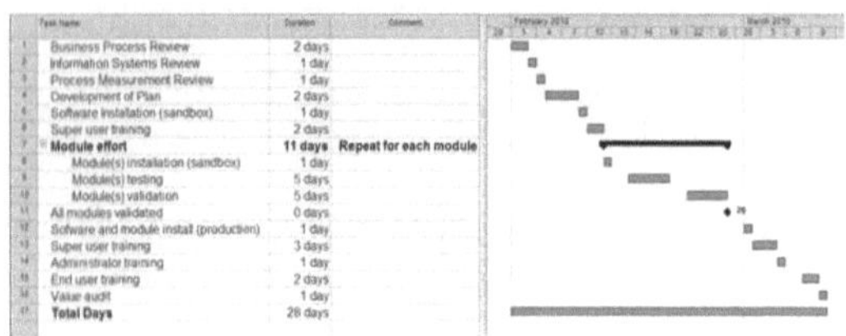

It's nice to read about all these concepts, but how can you really apply them to your own life?

This is what the chapter on implementation is all about, and it helps you plan a lifelong change in your health focus to live these principles and truly experience long term health, greater happiness, and extended longevity.

For five years I amended and improved these materials which now include a lot more information and helpful concepts for students wanting to improve their longevity and those of others.

I transcribed my videos and other materials to this book so you can read it all, and later hear it in an AudioBook.

This book is priced pretty inexpensively, compared to the online training and certification program which sells in total for $1,995 USD. If you are interested in taking the entire online program at a major discount, then please contact me at:

Marty@personal-longevity.com

Hope you enjoy these materials since when applied correctly they will significantly change your life.

PLP Concepts Overview

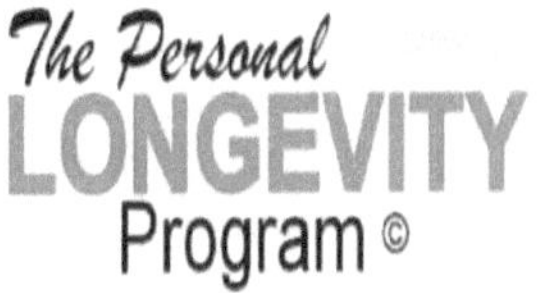

(Transcription of overview video)

Hello I'm Martin Ettington and I'd like to introduce you to the Personal Longevity Program which is an integrated holistic approach to long-term health. In this video we will only cover the high level concepts which comprise individual courses in the coaching certificate program for personal longevity.

The first concept is that long lived people exist and have existed for hundreds of thousands of years. We cover in the first course all about their records; along with people not only in places you might think like India, but in Europe and the United States-people who've lived long lives and well documented cases.

We discuss people who have lived well over the age of 120 and even the case of a Chinaman who lived to 256 years old. Plus a lot of mythology about people who have lived even longer lives so you get an idea that extending your life much longer than we think is currently medically and scientifically possible is certainly something that can happen.

The second course's concept has to do with finding your souls purpose. The point of wanting to live a long life is to know what your purpose in life is, so we go through some readings and some exercises to help you determine where soul's purpose in life is. Then doing goals as a fundamental concept so you will know the motivations in your life.

Third is the "Psychology of Living" also known by certain practitioners as "Removing the death Urge". The psychology of living has to do with seeking a positive image about your ability to live a long time. We tend to be programmed from birth about the idea that we are going to go through certain stages in our life as a child, as a teenager, and as adults. It's about reprogramming your subconscious as to the possibilities of a long life.

I've also learned in my life that it is very important to be able open your heart to unconditional love. When you're able to love unconditionally it also helps increase the strength of your immune system and fight off disease. So this is an aspect of spiritual growth. The courses also cover unconditional love and energy body forces. Managing your energy body is an important component of who you are in having energy working properly in your body and is another aspect of health for the length of longevity.

There are many types of scientific and medical research which are being done today and which will contribute to human longevity in the future.

Do you know that the average lifespan in the United States in 1900 was only about 40 years? We have doubled lifespan in the last century with current technologies but things under way in terms of scientific and medical improvements will help extend your lives further.

Also in this course on longevity we will cover a lot of the concepts which are being researched by scientists today. There are suggestions for more things you can do to do to use this science to improve your health along with physical supplements.

A unique thing that I thought about and decided to offer in these courses has to do with all my experiences in prophecy and how I was able to change outcomes on accidents that would occur to me by using simple exercises you can learn to change these outcomes. If you're in great health often the biggest thing you have to worry about are accidents.

We also provide guidelines you can follow on a daily basis and plans you can make to live healthier and happier and have a much longer life than you ever thought possible.

Thank you for listening !

Longevity Training-Book 7-The Science of Longevity

Course #7 Intro Video

(Transcription of Video)

Hello this is Marty Ettington and this is course number seven called the "Science of Longevity" about science and medical research into helping people live longer.

Even though this ten course program which is called the "Personal Longevity Coaching Program" is mainly about spiritual vital forces and what you can do to help improve your long-term health and lengthen your life. This program is a thorough holistic program on longevity. Without knowing something about what science and medicine are researching having to do with extending the human lifespan-let's go into a little history.

First of all if you look at actuarial statistics and historical records you'll find out that the average life expectancy in the United States in 1900 was only 30 to 40 years old. Which is short compared to today. Today's life spans are double. Back then if you think about the advances in medicine and nutrition everything-what would the life span of the average person-be by the end of the century by year 2100 could well be double again. So all my work is geared towards helping you live to at least 150 years and beyond.

And this is well within the realm of possibility given the advances on medical and scientific research. Everything I teach is really just in addition to your long-term health, happiness, and to increase your lifespan. In addition to all of that work-in this course we'll study several things.

One of the things we'll study is the longevity in plants and animals since they are our fellow genetic brothers here on this earth and we can learn a lot from them about their life spans, about the diets they have, about their lifestyles, and what causes them to be able to live to tremendous ages, I mean there are plants and trees that live to thousands of years, and animals that normally live to hundreds of years. So what is it about their makeup that we can learn that will help us extend our lives?

Another area we'll look at is what are current scientific research trends into improving human lifespan? These include things like the study of the chemical "Resveratrol's" role which is obtained from red wine grapes. And did you know that drinking red wine and actually helps to improve your life span?

Another is calorie restriction diets which have been shown in rats to help lengthen their lives. And calorie restriction in humans is thought now to help lengthen your life.

Telomeres are the end caps of different chromosomes in our body-in our cells. And these telomeres get shorter the older the cells are-so if there's a way to limit the degradation of telomeres that can increase lifespan. In other areas immortal cell lines having to do with cells that are basically immortal-and why is that? And how can that technology be applied to the knowledge of increasing our lifespan?

There are several other things too but the idea is to introduce you to current scientific and medical thought and then one of the assignments also within this course is a little bit of an overview.

If you don't already have any of my approaches of integration of the spirit and the energy body in the physical body and how that helps keep you healthy. And living a long time and how that integrates with scientific and medical research. So I hope you enjoy the course thank you very much.

Book-The Science of Longevity

Introduction to the Science of Longevity

Most of my books having to do with Longevity are focused on Spiritual and Vital forces related concepts and processes.

It's easy to forget that our life expectancy has doubled in the last one hundred years due to improved nutrition, medicine, and scientific breakthroughs.

No study or course on human longevity would be complete without learning about the conventional sides of science and medicine which can help our long term health and longevity.

Several mainstream authors have even written recently that over the next few decades our lifespans should have the potential for topping one hundred years on average—and this is without all the benefits of spiritual and vital forces practices.

At the end of this Ebook I've added a Chapter about the Personal Longevity Program which is one way to learn all about how to improve your long term health, happiness, and longevity by integrating Spirit, Mind, and Body.

It's a short description of what you will find on my site at
http://personal-longevity.com

The increase in Life Expectancy

Life expectancy is the average number of years a human has before death. It is conventionally calculated from the time of birth, but also can be calculated from any specified age.

For the past 150 years, best-performance life-expectancy (i.e. life-expectancy in the country where it is hi (recent Developments in the Ethics, Science, and Politics of Life-Extension, 2013-ghest) has increased at a very steady rate of 3 months per year. Life-expectancy for the ancient Romans was circa 23 years; today the average life-expectancy in the world is 64 years. Will this trend continue? What are the consequences if it does? And what ethical and political challenges does the prospect of life-extension create for us today? This article comments on some views on the ethics, science, and politics of life-extension from a recent edited volume, *The Fountain of Youth*.

Advances in sanitation, nutrition, and medical knowledge have made possible incredible changes in life expectancy throughout the world; providing subjects for study as well as the need to study them. In the United States, only 50 percent of children born in 1900 were expected to reach the age of 50; life expectancy today is approximately 83 years of age.

But note that there is a significant difference between male and female life expectancy - 82 years for men and 85 years for women. Life expectancy is lower for African Americans; 67.2 years for men and 74.7 years for women (Hoyert, Kochanek, and Murphy, 1999).

Life expectancy increased dramatically in the 20th century. These changes are the result of a combination of factors including nutrition, public health, and medicine only marginally. The most important single factor in the increase is the reduction of death in infancy.

The greatest improvements have been in the richest parts of the world. Life expectancy at birth in the United States in 1900 was 47 years. Life expectancy in India at mid-century was around 32; by 2000 it had risen to 64 years. According to the 2006 World Health Organization Report, due to HIV/AIDS and other health related issues today's life expectancy in poorer nations is almost half that of the industrialized, richer nations.

You will be able to see in below that for most of human history life expectancy was only 20-30 years old. What we would now consider young adulthood.

It was only in the early 20th Century that the average life length went up to 40 years.

The number of today's Octogenarians would be considered amazing and mostly unbelievable to people living 100 years ago.

Today's average world life expectancy of 66 years seems low to many of us raised in Western Countries.

Is it really that much more farfetched to be discussing how to double our present lifespans from today, considering that they have been doubled in the last 100 years?

The below Table shows how general life expectancy has changed in the world over millennia:

Humans by Era	Average Lifespan at Birth (years)
Neanderthal	20
Upper Paleolithic	33
Neolithic	20
Bronze Age[6]	18
Classical Greece[7]	20-30
Classical Rome[8][9]	20-30
Pre-Columbian North America[10]	25-35
Medieval Britain[11][12]	20-30
Early 20th Century[13][14]	30-40
Current world average[15][16]	66.12 (2008 est.)

Life Expectancy around the world today is shown below:

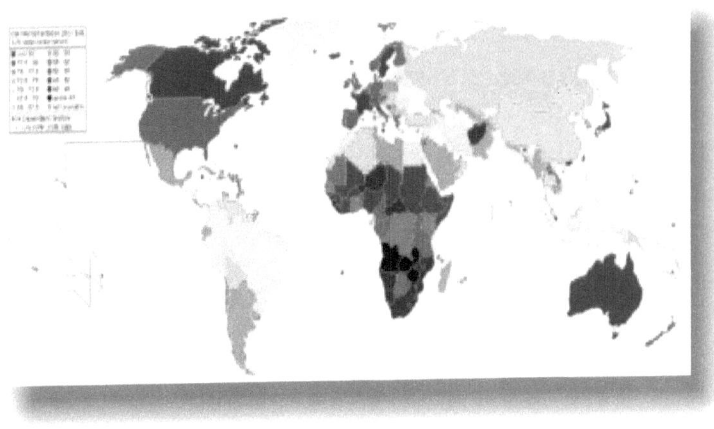

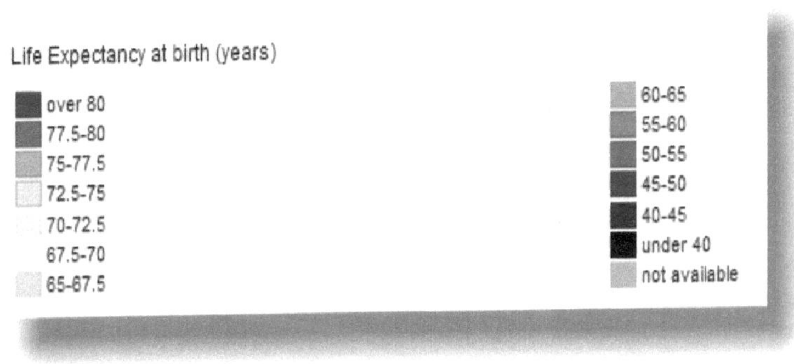

Much work is being done in Science today which may end up increasing our life expectancy significantly.

Long Lived Plants

One of the reasons to look at long lived plants and animals is because they have a similar genetic make-up and heritage to ourselves. If these plants and animals can have such long lives then maybe it's not too strange for humanity to have similar potentials.

<u>Clonal colonies</u>
As with all long-lived plants and fungal species, no individual part of a clonal colony is alive (in the sense of active metabolism) for more than a very small fraction of the life of the entire clone. Some clonal colonies may be fully connected via their root systems; while most are not actually interconnected, but are genetically identical clones which populate an area through vegetative reproduction.

Ages for clonal colonies, often based on current growth rates, are estimates:

- A huge colony of the sea grass Posidonia Oceanica in the Mediterranean Sea could be up to 100,000 years old.

- Pando (tree). This clonal colony of Populus Tremuloides has been estimated at 80,000 years old, although some claims place it as being as old as one million years.

- King's Lomatia in Tasmania: The sole surviving clonal colony of this species is estimated to be at least 43,600 years old.

- A huckleberry bush in Pennsylvania is thought to be as much as 13,000 years old.

- Eucalyptus Recurva: Clones in Australia are claimed to be 13,000 years old.

- Creosote bush: A ring of bushes in the Mojave Desert are estimated at 11,700 years of age.

- An individual of the fungus species Armillaria Ostoyae in the Malheur National Forest is thought to be between 2,000 and 8,500 years old. It is thought to be the world's largest organism by area, at 2,384 acres (965 hectares).

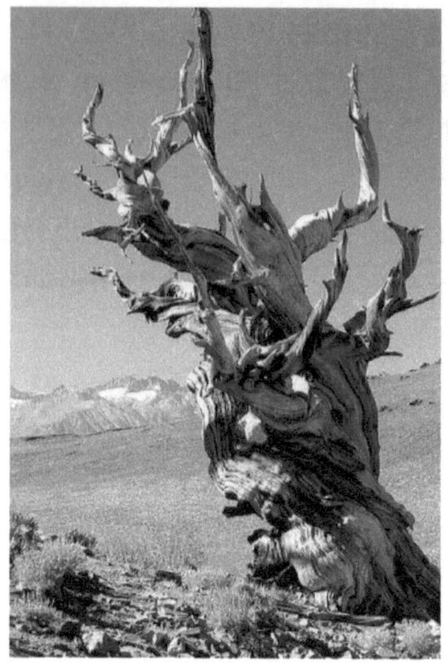

Individual plant specimens

- A cluster of Norway spruce in Sweden includes roots that have been carbon dated to 9,550 years old, which would make them the oldest known trees in the world! Individual tree trunks only last up to about 600   years, but the roots from which they grow have survived throughout the entire period.

- A Great Basin Bristlecone Pine (Pinus Longaeva) called Prometheus was measured by ring count at 4,862 years old when it was felled in 1964. This is the greatest verified age for any living organism at this time. Another great basin Bristlecone Pine, known as Methuselah, measured by ring count of sample cores is, at 4,838 years old, the oldest known tree in North America, and the oldest known individual tree in the world. (See picture above)

- Fortingall Yew, an ancient yew (Taxus Baccata) in the churchyard of the village of Fortingall in Perthshire, Scotland; is possibly the oldest known individual tree in Europe. Various estimates have put its age at between 2000 and 5000 years.

- Fitzroya Cupressoides is the species with the second oldest verified age, a specimen in Chile being measured by ring count as 3,622 years old.

- A Sacred Fig (Ficus Religiosa) specimen, the Sri Maha Bodhi, is (if its reported planting date of 288 BC is correct) at 2,293 years old, is the oldest known flowering plant.

- A specimen of Lagarostrobos Franklinii in Tasmania is thought to be about 2000 years old.

- Numerous Olive trees are purported to be 2000 years old or older. An olive tree in Crete, claiming such longevity, has been confirmed on the basis of tree ring analysis.

Long Lived Animals

You may be as surprised as I was to turn up all these records on long lived animals on our planet. If they can life so long why can't we eventually learn to do so?

- The Hydrozoan species Turritopsis nutricula is capable of cycling from a mature adult stage to an immature polyp stage and back again, indefinitely. This means there is, theoretically, no limit to its life span. Although no single specimen has been observed for any extended period   and it is impossible to estimate the age of a specimen.

- The Antarctic sponge Cinachyra Antarctica has an extremely slow   growth rate in the low temperatures of the Antarctic Ocean. One   specimen has been estimated to be 1,550 years old.

- A specimen of the Icelandic Cyprine Arctica Islandica (also known as an ocean Quahog), a mollusk, was found to have lived 405 years and   possibly up to 410. Another specimen had a recorded lifespan of 374 years.

- Some Koi fish have reportedly lived up to over 200 years, the oldest being Hanko; which died at an age of 215 years on July 7, 1977.

- Some unconfirmed sources estimated Bowhead whales to have lived up to 210 years of age. If proven this would make them the oldest mammals.

- Specimens of the Red Sea Urchin, Strongylocentrotus Franciscanus, have been found to be over 200 years old.

- Tu'i Malila, a radiated tortoise, died at an age of 188 years in May 1965. Harriet, a Galápagos tortoise died at an unconfirmed age of 175 years in June 2006.

- Timothy, a Greek tortoise, died at an age of 160 years in April 2004.

- Geoduck, a species of saltwater clam native to the Puget Sound, have been known to live over 160 years.

- A 109-year old female Blue-and-yellow Macaw named Charlie was hatched in 1899. It was incorrectly claimed that she formerly belonged to Winston Churchill.

- There is anecdotal evidence that the Patagonian tooth fish and sturgeon can live for over 100 years.

- The deep-sea hydrocarbon seep tubeworm Lamellibrachia Luymesi (Annelida, Polychaeta) lives for over 170 years.

Types of Biological Immortality

This can be defined as the absence of a sustained increase in rate of mortality as a function of chronological age. A cell or organism that does not experience, aging, is biologically immortal. However this definition of immortality was challenged in the "Handbook of the Biology of Aging", because the increase in rate of mortality as a function of chronological age may be negligible at extremely old ages (late-life mortality plateau). But even though the rate of mortality ceases to increase in old age, those rates are very high (e.g., 50% chance of surviving another year at age 110 or 115 years of age).

There is no known organism or individual cell that is inviolably immortal. Any life enjoying *biological immortality* can die if exposed to a toxic environment, or otherwise killed or destroyed.

<u>Cell lines</u>
Biologists have chosen the word immortal to designate cells that are not limited by the Hayflick limit (where cells no longer divide because of DNA damage or shortened telomeres). Prior to the work of Leonard Hayflick there was the erroneous belief fostered by Alexis Carrel that all normal somatic cells are immortal. (19)

The term immortalization was first applied to cancer cells that expressed the telomere lengthening enzyme telomerase, and thereby avoided apoptosis (programmed cell death). Among the most commonly used cell lines are

HeLa and Jurkat, both of which are immortalized cancer cells. Normal stem cells and germ cells can also be said to be immortal.

Immortal cell lines of cancer cells can be created by induction of oncogenes or loss of tumor suppressor genes. One way to induce immortality is through viral-mediated induction of the large T-antigen, commonly introduced through simian virus 40 (SV-40).

In terms of multi-cellular organisms, immortality may not be a desirable condition, as the main controls over cancer are the apoptotic mechanisms.

Bacteria
Bacteria can be said to be biologically immortal, but only as a colony. An individual bacterium can easily die. The two daughter bacteria resulting from cell division of a parent bacterium can be regarded as unique individuals or as embers of a biologically "immortal" colony. The two daughter cells can be regarded as "rejuvenated" copies of the parent cell because damaged macromolecules have been split between the two cells and diluted. In the same way stem cells and gametes can be regarded as "immortal".

Hydra
Hydras are a genus of simple, fresh-water animals possessing radial symmetry and no post-mitotic cells. The fact that all cells continually divide allows defects and toxins to be "diluted-away". It has been suggested that

hydras do not undergo senescence (aging), and so are biologically immortal.

Life Extension Technologies

Some life extensionists, such as those who practice cryonics, have the hope that humans may someday become biologically immortal. This would not be the same as literal immortality, since people can always be murdered or die in accidents. (Mind uploading, however, could allow literal immortality in a sense, by uploading backups into cloned or artificial bodies after an accident. See Mind uploading in science fiction.)

However, this practice may not actually allow for one to continue their life through the backup, and since two (or more) beings with identical minds have never existed before, it is unknown whether or not they could share consciousness on any level.

Nanotechnology

Nanotechnology, and specifically of nano-medicine, have recently increased awareness of the possibilities for biological immortality in humans. A study published in Physiological and Biochemical Zoology in 2005 indicates that biological immortality may exist in humans at a late stage in life: "the exponential increase in age-specific death rate seemed to slow down.

Future advances in nanomedicine could give rise to life extension through the repair of many processes thought to be responsible for aging. K. Eric Drexler, one of the founders of nanotechnology, postulated cell repair machines, including ones operating within cells and utilizing as yet hypothetical molecular computers, in his 1986 book Engines of Creation. Raymond Kurzweil, a futurist and transhumanist, stated in his book The Singularity Is Near that he believes that advanced medical nanorobotics could completely remedy the effects of aging by 2030.

Cloning and body part replacement

Some life extensionists suggest that therapeutic cloning and stem cell research could one day provide a way to generate cells, body parts, or even entire bodies (generally referred to as reproductive cloning) that would be genetically identical to a prospective patient. Recently, the US Department of Defense initiated a program to research the possibility of growing human body parts on mice. Complex biological structures, such as mammalian joints and limbs, have not yet been replicated. Dog and primate brain transplantation experiments were conducted in the mid-20th century but failed due to rejection and the inability to restore nerve connections. As of 2006, the implantation of bio-engineered bladders grown from patients' own cells has proven to be a viable treatment for bladder disease.[25] Proponents of body part replacement and cloning contend that the required biotechnologies are likely to appear earlier than other life-extension technologies.

The use of human stem cells, particularly embryonic stem cells, is controversial. Opponents' objections generally are based on interpretations of religious teachings or ethical considerations. Proponents of stem cell research point out that cells are routinely formed and destroyed in a variety of contexts. Use of stem cells taken from the umbilical cord or parts of the adult body may not provoke controversy.

The controversies over cloning are similar, except general public opinion in most countries stands in opposition to reproductive cloning. Some proponents of therapeutic cloning predict the production of whole bodies, lacking consciousness, for eventual brain transplantation.

Cryonics

For cryonicists (advocates of cryopreservation), storing the body at low temperatures after death may provide an "ambulance" into a future in which advanced medical technologies may allow resuscitation and repair. They speculate cryogenic temperatures will minimize changes in biological tissue for many years, giving the medical community ample time to cure all disease, rejuvenate the aged and repair any damage that is caused by the cryopreservation process.

Many cryonicists do not believe that legal death is "real death" because stoppage of heartbeat and breathing—the usual medical criteria for legal death—occur before biological death of cells and tissues of the body. Even at room temperature, cells may take hours to die and days to decompose. Although neurological damage occurs within

4–6 minutes of cardiac arrest, the irreversible neurodegenerative processes do not manifest for hours. Cryonicist's state that rapid cooling and cardio-pulmonary support applied immediately after certification of death can preserve cells and tissues for long-term preservation at cryogenic temperatures. People, particularly children, have survived up to an hour without heartbeat after submersion in ice water. In one case, full recovery was reported after 45 minutes underwater. To facilitate rapid preservation of cells and tissue, cryonics "standby teams" are available to wait by the bedside of patients who are to be cryopreserved to apply cooling and cardio-pulmonary support as soon as possible after declaration of death.

No mammal has been successfully cryopreserved and brought back to life, and resuscitation from cryonics is not possible with current science. Some scientists still support the idea based on their expectations of the capabilities of future science.

Red Wine Extract- Resvesterol

The groups of Howitz and Sinclair reported in 2003 in the journal, Nature, that resveratrol significantly extends the lifespan of the yeast Saccharomyces cerevisiae.Later studies conducted by Sinclair showed that resveratrol also prolongs the lifespan of the worm, Caenorhabditis elegans, and the fruit fly, Drosophila melanogaster. In 2007, a different group of researchers were able to reproduce Sinclair's results with C. elegans, but a third group could not achieve consistent increases in lifespan of either D. melanogaster or C. elegans.

In 2006, Italian scientists obtained the first positive result of resveratrol supplementation in a vertebrate. Using a short-lived fish, Nothobranchius furzeri, with a median life span of nine weeks. They found a maximal dose of resveratrol increased the median lifespan by 56%. Compared with the control fish at nine weeks, that is, by the end of control fish's life, the fish supplemented with resveratrol showed significantly higher swimming activity and better learning to avoid an unpleasant stimulus. The authors noted a slight increase of mortality in young fish caused by resveratrol, and hypothesized that its weak toxic action stimulated the defense mechanisms and resulted in the life span extension.

Later the same year, Sinclair reported resveratrol counteracted the detrimental effects of a high-fat diet in mice. The high-fat diet was compounded by adding hydrogenated coconut oil to the standard diet; it provided

60% of energy from fat, and the mice on it consumed about 30% more calories than the mice on standard diet and became obese and diabetic. Mice on the high-fat diet exhibited a high mortality rate compared to mice fed the standard diet; mice fed the high-fat diet plus 22 mg/kg resveratrol had a 30% lower risk of death than the mice on the high-fat diet alone, making their death rates similar to those on the standard diet. The supplement also partially corrected a subset of the abnormal gene expression profile and abnormal insulin and glucose metabolism. Resveratrol supplements did not change the levels of free fatty acids and cholesterol, however, which were much higher than in the mice on standard diet.

A further study by a group of scientists, which included Sinclair, indicated resveratrol treatment had a range of beneficial effects in elderly mice, but did not increase the longevity of ad libitum–fed (freely-feeding) mice when started midlife. Later, the National Institute on Aging's Interventions Testing Program (ITP) also tested three different doses of resveratrol in mice on a normal diet beginning in young adulthood, and again found no effect on lifespan, even at doses roughly eight times higher than those that had normalized the lifespan of the high-fat-fed, obese mice in the earlier study.

A 2011 study published in Nature suggested that some of the benefits demonstrated in previous studies were overrepresented, however, this study was challenged immediately, and few experiments were suggested to be of inferior quality.

Johan Auwerx (at the Institute of Genetics and Molecular and Cell Biology in Illkirch, France) and coauthors published an online article in the journal Cell in November 2006. Mice fed resveratrol for fifteen weeks had better treadmill endurance than controls. The study supported Sinclair's hypothesis that the effects of resveratrol are indeed due to the activation of the Sirtuin 1 gene.

Nicholas Wade's interview-article with Dr. Auwerx stated the dose was 400 mg/kg of body weight (much higher than the 22 mg/kg of the Sinclair study). For an 80 kg (175 lb) person, the 400 mg/kg of body weight amount used in Auwerx's mouse study would total 30,000 mg/day. Compensating for the fact that humans have slower metabolic rates than mice would change the equivalent human dose to roughly 4000 mg/day. Again, there is no published evidence anywhere in the scientific literature of any clinical trial for efficacy in humans. There are limited human safety data. Long-term safety has not been evaluated in humans.

In a study of 123 Finnish adults, those born with certain increased variations of the SIRT1 gene had faster metabolisms, helping them to burn more energy, indicating the same pathway shown in the laboratory mice works in humans.

Calorie Restriction Diets

In human subjects, CR has been shown to lower cholesterol, fasting glucose, and blood pressure. Some consider these to be biomarkers of aging, since there is a correlation between these markers and risk of diseases associated with aging. Except for houseflies, animal species tested with CR so far, including primates, rats, mice, spiders, *Drosophila*, *C. Elegans* and rotifers, have shown lifespan extension. CR is the only known dietary measure capable of extending maximum lifespan, as opposed to average lifespan. In CR, energy intake is minimized, but sufficient quantities of vitamins, minerals and other important nutrients must be eaten.

In the US at the Washington University School of Medicine in St. Louis a small scale study showing the effects of following a calorie restricted diet of 10-25% less calorie intake than the average Western diet. Body mass index (BMI) was significantly lower in the calorie-restricted group when compared with the matched group; 19.6 compared with 25.9. The BMI values for the comparison group are similar to the mean BMI values for middle-aged people in the US.

In 1934, Mary Crowell and Clive McCay of Cornell University observed that laboratory rats fed a severely reduced calorie diet while maintaining micronutrient levels resulted in life spans of up to twice as long as otherwise expected. These findings were explored in detail by a series of experiments with mice conducted by Roy Walford and his student Richard Weindruch. In 1986,

Weindruch reported that restricting the calorie intake of laboratory mice proportionally increased their life span compared to a group of mice with a normal diet. The calorie-restricted mice also maintained youthful appearances and activity levels longer and showed delays in age-related diseases. The results of the many experiments by Walford and Weindruch were summarized in their book The Retardation of Aging and Disease by Dietary Restriction (1988) (ISBN 0-398-05496-7).

The findings have since been accepted and generalized to a range of other animals. Researchers are investigating the possibility of parallel physiological links in humans. In the meantime, many people have independently adopted the practice of calorie restriction in some form.

In 1989, scientists at University of Wisconsin started a study of 20 adult male rhesus monkeys; 9 of them were put on a normal diet and 11 were subjected to a 30% reduction in dietary intake. Results are being periodically published.

A study at UCSF called "CRONA" was started in December 2010, and studied 28 long-term CR practitioners over a few months. The study was completed on September 20, 2011. As of August 2012 the results had not yet been published.

Hormone treatments

The anti-aging industry offers several hormone therapies. Some of these have been criticized for possible dangers to the patient and a lack of proven effect. For example, the American Medical Association has been critical of some anti-aging hormone therapies.

Even if some recent clinical studies have shown that low-dose GH treatment for adults with GH deficiency changes the body composition by increasing muscle mass, decreasing fat mass, increasing bone density and muscle strength, improves cardiovascular parameters (i.e. decrease of LDL cholesterol), and affects the quality of life without significant side effects. The evidence for use of growth hormone as an anti-aging therapy is mixed and based on animal studies. An early study suggested that supplementation of mice with growth hormone increased average life expectancy.[20] Additional animal experiments have suggested that growth hormone may generally act to shorten maximum lifespan; knockout mice lacking the receptor for growth hormone live especially long. Furthermore, mouse models lacking the insulin-like growth factor also live especially long and have low levels of growth hormone.

Insulinlike growth factor (IGF-1) restriction

People suffering from rare condition known as Laron syndrome have mutation in the gene that makes the receptor for growth hormone. It's theorized that that mutation may hold a key to life extension.

Dr. Longo said that some level of IGF-1 was necessary to protect against heart disease, but that lowering the level might be beneficial. A drug that does this is already on the market for treatment of acromegaly, a thickening of the bones caused by excessive growth hormone. "Our underlying hypothesis is that this drug would prolong life span," Dr. Longo said. He said he was not taking the drug, called pegvisomant or Somavert, which is very hard to obtain.

Antioxidants

Antioxidants are natural substances in foods. They may help protect you from disease by preventing the harmful effects of oxygen free radicals on your body. Oxygen free radicals are formed as cells in your body combine with oxygen to make energy. Free radicals also come from smoking or being exposed to things in the environment like radiation or sunlight. As we age, this damage may build up. According to one theory of aging, in time this build-up harms cells, tissues, and organs.

Your body's own antioxidant defense system stops most free-radical damage, but not all. Antioxidants may prevent cataracts and heart disease, protect against damage from smoking, or boost immunity to illness.

Some antioxidants, such as the enzyme SOD (superoxide dismutase), are only useful when produced in the body. SOD pills have no effect on the body. They are broken up into different substances during digestion. Other antioxidants that come from food include:

- beta-carotene, present in deep-colored fruits and vegetables,
- selenium, found in seafood, liver, meat, and grains
- vitamin C, from citrus fruits, peppers, tomatoes, and berries, and

- Vitamin E, present in wheat germ, nuts, sesame seeds, and canola, olive, and peanut oils.

How much of these anti-oxidants should you use, if at all? The National Academy of Sciences is a nongovernmental group of experts involved in scientific research. They recommend what vitamins and minerals you need in your diet and how much of each. They say that there is no proof that large doses of anti-oxidants will prevent chronic diseases such as heart disease, diabetes, or cataracts.

They did set guidelines for the safe use of some of them:

- Selenium-at least 55 micro-grams (mcg) per day but not more than 400 mcg per day.
- Vitamin C-at least 75 milligrams (mg) per day for women and 90 mg for men, although smokers need more. No one should have more than 2,000 mg per day.
- Vitamin E-at least 15 mg per day from food and not more than 1,000 mg per day.

Telomeres

A telomere is a region of repetitive DNA at the end of chromosomes, which protects the end of the chromosome from destruction. Its name is derived from the Greek nouns telos (τέλος) "end" and meros (μέρος, root: μερεσ-) "part".

During cell division, the enzymes that duplicate the chromosome and its DNA can't continue their duplication all the way to the end of the chromosome. If cells divided without telomeres, they would lose the end of their chromosomes, and the necessary information it contains. (In 1972, James Watson named this phenomenon the "end replication problem".)

The telomere is a disposable buffer, which is consumed during cell division and is replenished by an enzyme, the telomerase reverse transcriptase.

In 1975-1977, Elizabeth Blackburn, working as a postdoctoral fellow at Yale University with Joseph Gall, discovered the unusual nature of telomeres, with their simple repeated DNA sequences composing chromosome ends. Their work was published in 1978.

This mechanism usually limits cells to a fixed number of divisions, and animal studies suggest that this is responsible for aging on the cellular level and affects lifespan. Telomeres protect a cell's chromosomes from fusing with each other or rearranging.

These chromosome abnormalities can lead to cancer, so cells are normally destroyed when telomeres are consumed. Most cancer is the result of cells bypassing the Telomere destruction. Biologists speculate that this mechanism is a tradeoff between aging and cancer.

Some scientists think that by finding a way to lengthen the telomeres in our cells we wouldn't have as much cell damage when cells replicate, and therefore live much longer lives.

Electronic, Digital, and Technological Solutions

One area of life extension I'm not addressing in this book is what you might call the technological solution.

These are solutions to download consciousness into computers or provide backup computing power to manage consciousness and memories.

My problem with this approach is that since I strongly believe that all of us have an immortal soul which is separate from our physical bodies. Therefore, any type of currently envisioned technological storage approach would only store a portion of the physical mind-not any elements of the Spirit.

Summary of The Science of Longevity

There are a variety of scientific and medical ideas on human life extension.

The amount of thought which has been put into this subject shows how important life extension is to the whole human race.

This book doesn't list every possible scientific or medical idea for life extension, but it does review the most popular and most potentially exciting ones.

Even though most of what I write has to do with life extension from "Spiritual and Vital forces approaches-I'm open minded to the idea of using whatever concepts, techniques, and approaches which work.

Maybe the ideal approach is to choose a combination of all types of concepts, processes, and techniques for individual life extension—with the individual in charge of choosing what approaches they will use to improve their long term health and longevity.

Science Articles on Longevity

Below is a series of articles about discoveries on longevity from scientific research:

Gene Variant Linked to Active Personality Traits Also Linked to Human Longevity

Jan. 3, 2013 — A variant of a gene associated with active personality traits in humans seems to also be involved with living a longer life, UC Irvine and other researchers have found.

This derivative of a dopamine-receptor gene -- called the DRD4 7R allele -- appears in significantly higher rates in people more than 90 years old and is linked to lifespan increases in mouse studies.

Robert Moyzis, professor of biological chemistry at UC Irvine, and Dr. Nora Volkow, a psychiatrist who conducts research at the Brookhaven National Laboratory and also directs the National Institute on Drug Abuse, led a research effort that included data from the UC Irvine-led 90+ Study in Laguna Woods, Calif. Results appear online in *The Journal of Neuroscience*.

The variant gene is part of the dopamine system, which facilitates the transmission of signals among neurons and plays a major role in the brain network responsible for attention and reward-driven learning. The DRD4 7R allele blunts dopamine signaling, which enhances individuals' reactivity to their environment.

People who carry this variant gene, Moyzis said, seem to be more motivated to pursue social, intellectual and physical activities. The variant is also linked to attention-deficit/hyperactivity disorder and addictive and risky behaviors.

"While the genetic variant may not directly influence longevity," Moyzis said, "it is associated with personality traits that have been shown to be important for living a longer, healthier life. It's been well documented that the more you're involved with social and physical activities, the more likely you'll live longer. It could be as simple as that." Numerous studies -- including a number from the 90+ Study -- have confirmed that being active is important for successful aging, and it may deter the advancement of neurodegenerative diseases, such as Alzheimer's.

Prior molecular evolutionary research led by Moyzis and Chuansheng Chen, UC Irvine professor of psychology & social behavior, indicated that this "longevity allele" was selected for during the nomadic out-of-Africa human exodus more than 30,000 years ago.

In the new study, the UC Irvine team analyzed genetic samples from 310 participants in the 90+ Study. This "oldest-old" population had a 66 percent increase in individuals carrying the variant relative to a control group of 2,902 people between the ages of 7 and 45. The presence of the variant also was strongly correlated with higher levels of physical activity.

Next, Volkow, neuroscientist Panayotis Thanos and their colleagues at the Brookhaven National Laboratory found that mice without the variant had a 7 percent to 9.7 percent decrease in lifespan compared with those possessing the gene, even when raised in an enriched environment.

While it's evident that the variant can contribute to longevity, Moyzis said further studies must take place to identify any immediate clinical benefits from the research. "However, it is clear that individuals with this gene variant are already more likely to be responding to the well-known medical adage to get more physical activity," he added.

Genetic Signatures of Exceptional Longevity

Jan. 18, 2012 — While environment and family history are factors in healthy aging, genetic variants play a critical and complex role in conferring exceptional longevity, according to researchers from the Boston University Schools of Public Health and Medicine, Boston Medical Center, IRCCS Multimedica in Milan, Italy, and Yale University. Published in *PLoS ONE*, after peer review, the research findings are the corrected version of work originally published in *Science* in July 2010. The revised publication includes additional authors who independently assessed and helped to produce a valid genotype data set, for which the same analysis as in the original paper was performed. It also contains an additional replication data set of subjects with an average age of 107.

Centenarians are a model of healthy aging, as the onset of disability in these individuals is generally delayed until they are well into their mid-90s. Because exceptional longevity can run strongly in families, and numerous animal studies have suggested a strong genetic influence on life span, the researchers set out to determine which genetic variants play roles in human survival beyond 100 years of age. They used a well-established Bayesian statistical method for determining which single nucleotide polymorphisms (SNPs, or genetic variants) could, as a group, be used to categorize subjects as centenarians versus controls, based solely upon the genetic information. The predictive sensitivity of the model they developed, which contains 281 SNPs, increased with the age of the subject, supporting the hypothesis that genes play an increasingly strong role in survival in centenarians.

The model was able to predict exceptional longevity with 60 to 85 percent accuracy, depending on the average age of the replication sample that was used. The older the sample, the stronger the sensitivity. Many of the 130 known genes associated with the SNPs in the prediction model have been shown by other gerontologists to play roles in age-related diseases and aging, said the study's lead researchers, Paola Sebastiani, PhD, professor of biostatistics at the BU School of Public Health, and Thomas Perls, MD, MPH, associate professor of medicine at the BU School of Medicine.

"This is a useful step towards meaningful predictive medicine and personal genomics," said Dr. Perls, a geriatrician at Boston Medical Center. "When people can do this kind of analysis on whole genome sequences for traits that have important genetic components, the predictive value should be even better."

The new study differs from the earlier study, voluntarily retracted by the authors, in several ways: A select group of faulty SNPs was eliminated from this study; an additional sample of extremely old study subjects was added; and researchers from Yale University were called in to independently validate the data and methodology. The corrected study, as did the original, found that subjects who shared the same profile of variations for genetic markers in the model appeared to share similar levels of risk for various traits or diseases associated with exceptional longevity -- most notably, in their ages of survival. "Further study of these genetic characteristics may yield a better understanding of the genetic and biological bases of delaying or escaping age-related diseases and achieving longer survival," Dr. Perls said. "The novel approach to genetic data that is described here is likely applicable to other complex inherited traits, and we look forward to other research groups applying these methods to their data."

Low Vitamin D Levels Linked to Longevity, Surprising Study Shows

Nov. 5, 2012 — Low levels of vitamin D may be associated with longevity, according to a study involving middle-aged children of people in their 90s published in *CMAJ* (*Canadian Medical Association Journal*).

"We found that familial longevity was associated with lower levels of vitamin D and a lower frequency of allelic variation in the CYP2R1 gene, which was associated with higher levels of vitamin D," writes Dr. Diana van Heemst, Department of Gerontology and Geriatrics, Leiden University Medical Center, Leiden, the Netherlands, with coauthors.

Previous studies have shown that low levels of vitamin D are associated with increased rates of death, heart disease, diabetes, cancer, allergies, mental illness and other afflictions. However, it is not known whether low levels are the cause of these diseases or if they are a consequence.

To determine whether there was an association between vitamin D levels and longevity, Dutch researchers looked at data from 380 white families with at least 2 siblings over age 90 (89 years or older for men and 91 year or older for women) in the Leiden Longevity Study. The study involved the siblings, their offspring and their offspring's partners for a total of 1038 offspring and 461 controls. The children of the nonagenarians were included because it is difficult to include controls for the older age group. The partners were included because they were of a similar age and shared similar environmental factors that might influence vitamin D levels.

The researchers measured levels of 25(OH) vitamin D and categorized levels by month as they varied according to season. Tanning bed use, which can affect vitamin D levels, was categorized as never, 1 times per year and 6 times per year. The researchers controlled for age, sex, BMI (body mass index), time of year, vitamin supplementation and kidney function, all factors that can influence vitamin D levels. They also looked at the influence of genetic variation in 3 genes associated with vitamin D levels.

"We found that the offspring of nonagenarians who had at least 1 nonagenarian sibling had lower levels of vitamin D than controls, independent of possible confounding factors and SNPs [single nucleotide polymorphisms] associated with vitamin D levels," write the authors. "We also found that the offspring had a lower frequency of common genetic variants in the CYP2R1 gene; a common genetic variant of this gene predisposes people to high vitamin D levels.

Why Some Animals Live Longer Than Others

Mar. 29, 2012 — Scientists at the University of Liverpool have developed a new method to detect proteins associated with longevity, which helps further our understanding into why some animals live longer than others.

The team looked at the genome of more than 30 mammalian species to identify proteins that evolve in connection with the longevity of a species. They found that a protein, important in responding to DNA damage, evolves and mutates in a non-random way in species that are longer-lived, suggesting that it is changing for a specific purpose. They found a similar pattern in proteins associated with metabolism, cholesterol and pathways involved in the recycling of proteins.

Findings show that if certain proteins are being selected by evolution to change in long-lived mammals like humans and elephants, then it is possible that these species have optimized pathways that repair molecular damage, compared to shorter-lived animals, such as mice.
The study, led by Dr Joao Pedro Magalhaes and postgraduate student, Yang Li, is the first to show evolutionary patterns in biological repair systems in long-lived animals and could, in the future, be used to help develop anti-aging interventions by identifying proteins in long-lived species that better respond to, for example, DNA damage. Proteins associated with the degradation of damaged proteins, a process that has been connected to aging, were also linked with the evolution of longevity in mammals.

Dr Magalhaes, from the University's Institute of Integrative Biology, said: "The genetic basis for longevity differences between species remains a major puzzle of biology. A mouse lives less than five years and yet humans can live to over 100 for example. If we can identify the proteins that allow some species to live longer than others we could use this knowledge to improve human health and slow the aging process.

"We developed a method to detect proteins whose molecular evolution correlates with longevity of a species. The proteins we detected changed in a particular pattern, suggesting that evolution of these proteins was not by accident, but rather by design to cope with the biological processes impacted by aging, such as DNA damage. The results suggest that long-lived animals were able to optimise bodily repair which will help them fend off the aging process."

The research is published in the American Aging Association's journal, *Age*.

How Calorie-Restricted Diets Fight Obesity and Extend Life Span

Dec. 29, 2009 — Scientists searching for the secrets of how calorie-restricted diets increase longevity are reporting discovery of proteins in the fat cells of human volunteers that change as pounds drop off. The proteins could become markers for monitoring or boosting the effectiveness of calorie-restricted diets -- the only scientifically proven way of extending life span in animals. Their study appears online in ACS' *Journal of Proteome Research*.

Edwin Mariman and colleagues note that scientists have long known that sharply restricting intake of calories while maintaining good nutrition makes animals live longer and stay healthier. Recent studies suggest that people may gain similar benefits. But scientists know little about how these diets work in humans, particularly their effects on cells that store fat.

The new study focused on proteins in abdominal subcutaneous fat cells from a group of overweight people before and after they went on a five-week-long calorie-restricted diet. The volunteers each lost an average of 21 pounds. Scientists identified changes in the levels of 6 proteins as the volunteers shed pounds, including proteins that tell the body to store fat. These proteins could serve as important markers for improving or tracking the effectiveness of therapies involving calorie-restricted diets, they say.

Key Genes That Switch Off With Aging Highlighted as Potential Targets for Anti-Aging Therapies

Apr. 19, 2012 — Researchers have identified key genes that switch off with aging, highlighting them as potential targets for anti-aging therapies.

Researchers at King's College London, in collaboration with the Wellcome Trust Sanger Institute, have identified a group of 'aging' genes that are switched on and off by natural mechanisms called epigenetic factors, influencing the rate of healthy aging and potential longevity.

The study also suggests these epigenetic processes -- that can be caused by external factors such as diet, lifestyle and environment -- are likely to be initiated from an early age and continue through a person's life. The researchers say that the epigenetic changes they have identified could be used as potential 'markers' of biological aging and in the future could be possible targets for anti-aging therapies. Published April 20 in *PLoS Genetics*, the study looked at 172 twins aged 32 to 80 from the TwinsUK cohort based at King's College London and St Thomas' Hospital, as part of King's Health Partners Academic Health Sciences Centre.

The researchers looked for epigenetic changes in the twins' DNA, and performed epigenome-wide association scans to analyze these changes in relation to chronological age. They identified 490 age related epigenetic changes. They also analysed DNA modifications in age related traits and found that epigenetic changes in four genes relate to cholesterol, lung function and maternal longevity.

To try to identify when these epigenetic changes may be triggered, the researchers replicated the study in 44 younger twins, aged 22 to 61, and found that many of the 490 age related epigenetic changes were also present in this younger group. The researchers say these results suggest that while many age related epigenetic changes happen naturally with age throughout a person's life, a proportion of these changes may be initiated early in life. Dr Jordana Bell from King's College London, who co-led the study said: 'We found that epigenetic changes associate with age related traits that have previously been used to define biological age.

'We identified many age-related epigenetic changes, but four seemed to impact the rate of healthy aging and potential longevity and we can use these findings as potential markers of aging. These results can help understand the biological mechanisms underlying healthy aging and age-related disease, and future work will explore how environmental effects can affect these epigenetic changes.'

Dr Panos Deloukas, co-leader of the study from the Wellcome Trust Sanger Institute, said: 'Our study interrogated only a fraction of sites in the genome that carry such epigenetic changes; these initial findings support the need for a more comprehensive scan of epigenetic variation.'

Professor Tim Spector, senior author from King's College London, said: 'This study is the first glimpse of the potential that large twin studies have to find the key genes involved in aging, how they can be modified by lifestyle and start to develop anti-aging therapies. The future will be very exciting for age research.'

'Personality Genes' May Help Account for Longevity

May 24, 2012 — "It's in their genes" is a common refrain from scientists when asked about factors that allow centenarians to reach age 100 and beyond. Up until now, research has focused on genetic variations that offer a physiological advantage such as high levels of HDL ("good") cholesterol. But researchers at Albert Einstein College of Medicine and Ferkauf Graduate School of Psychology of Yeshiva University have found that personality traits like being outgoing, optimistic, easygoing, and enjoying laughter as well as staying engaged in activities may also be part of the longevity genes mix. The findings, published online May 21 in the journal *Aging*, come from Einstein's Longevity Genes Project, which includes over 500 Ashkenazi Jews over the age of 95, and 700 of their offspring. Ashkenazi (Eastern European) Jews were selected because they are genetically homogeneous, making it easier to spot genetic differences within the study population.

Previous studies have indicated that personality arises from underlying genetic mechanisms that may directly affect health. The present study of 243 of the centenarians (average age 97.6 years, 75 percent women) was aimed at detecting genetically-based personality characteristics by developing a brief measure (the Personality Outlook Profile Scale, or POPS) of personality in centenarians.

"When I started working with centenarians, I thought we'd find that they survived so long in part because they were mean and ornery," said Nir Barzilai, M.D., the Ingeborg and Ira Leon Rennert Chair of Aging Research, director of Einstein's Institute for Aging Research and co-corresponding author of the study. "But when we assessed the personalities of these 243 centenarians, we found qualities that clearly reflect a positive attitude towards life. Most were outgoing, optimistic and easygoing. They considered laughter an important part of life and had a large social network. They expressed emotions openly rather than bottling them up." In addition, the centenarians had lower scores for displaying neurotic personality and higher scores for being conscientious compared with a representative sample of the U.S. population.

"Some evidence indicates that personality can change between the ages of 70 and 100, so we don't know whether our centenarians have maintained their personality traits across their entire lifespans," continued Dr. Barzilai. "Nevertheless, our findings suggest that centenarians share particular personality traits and that genetically-based aspects of personality may play an important role in achieving both good health and exceptional longevity."

Solving the Mystery of Aging: Longevity Gene Makes Hydra Immortal and Humans Grow Older

Nov. 13, 2012 — Why do we get older? When do we die and why? Is there a life without aging? For centuries, science has been fascinated by these questions. Now researchers from Kiel (Germany) have examined why the polyp Hydra is immortal -- and unexpectedly discovered a link to aging in humans.

The study carried out by Kiel University together with the University Medical Center Schleswig-Holstein (UKSH) will be published this week in the *Proceedings of the National Academy of Sciences* (PNAS).

Hydra -- mysteriously immortal

The tiny freshwater polyp Hydra does not show any signs of aging and is potentially immortal. There is a rather simple biological explanation for this: these animals exclusively reproduce by budding rather than by mating. A prerequisite for such vegetative-only reproduction is that each polyp contains stem cells capable of continuous proliferation. Without these stem cells, the animals could not reproduce any more. Due to its immortality, Hydra has been the subject of many studies regarding aging processes for several years.

Aging in humans

When people get older, more and more of their stem cells lose the ability to proliferate and thus to form new cells. Aging tissue cannot regenerate any more, which is why for example muscles decline. Elderly people tend to feel weaker because their heart muscles are affected by this aging process as well. If it were possible to influence these aging processes, humans could feel physically better for much longer. Studying animal tissue such as those of Hydra -- an animal full of active stem cells during all its life -- may deliver valuable insight into stem cell aging as such.

Human longevity gene discovered in Hydra

"Surprisingly, our search for the gene that causes Hydra to be immortal led us to the so-called FoxO gene," says Anna-Marei Böhm, PhD student and first author of the study. The FoxO gene exists in all animals and humans and has been known for years. However, until now it was not known why human stem cells become fewer and inactive with increasing age, which biochemical mechanisms are involved and if FoxO played a role in aging. In order to find the gene, the research group isolated Hydra's stem cells and then screened all of their genes.

Immortality mechanism of Hydra revealed

The Kiel research team examined FoxO in several genetically modified polyps: Hydra with normal FoxO, with inactive FoxO and with enhanced FoxO. The scientists were able to show that animals without FoxO possess significantly fewer stem cells. Interestingly, the immune system in animals with inactive FoxO also changes drastically. "Drastic changes of the immune system similar to those observed in Hydra are also known from elderly humans," explains Philip Rosenstiel of the Institute of Clinical Molecular Biology at UKSH, whose research group contributed to the study.

FoxO makes human life longer, too

"Our research group demonstrated for the first time that there is a direct link between the FoxO gene and aging," says Thomas Bosch from the Zoological Institute of Kiel University, who led the Hydra study. Bosch continues: "FoxO has been found to be particularly active in centenarians -- people older than one hundred years -- which is why we believe that FoxO plays a key role in aging -- not only in Hydra but also in humans." However, the hypothesis cannot be verified on humans, as this would require a genetic manipulation of humans. Bosch stresses however that the current results are still a big step forward in explaining how humans age. Therefore the next step must be to study how the longevity gene FoxO works in Hydra, and how environmental factors influence FoxO activity.

Without stem cells we all die

Scientifically, the study has two major conclusions: On the one hand it confirms that the FoxO gene plays a decisive role in the maintenance of stem cells. It thus determines the life span of animals -- from cnidarians to humans. On the other hand, the study shows that aging and longevity of organisms really depend on two factors: the maintenance of stem cells and the maintenance of a functioning immune system.

Spirituality Key to Chinese Medicine Success: Study Explores Why Chinese Medicine Has Stood the Test of Time

Sep. 25, 2012 — Are the longevity and vitality of traditional Chinese medicine (TCM) due to its holistic approach? Indeed, Chinese medicine is not simply about treating illness, but rather about taking care of the whole person -- body, mind, and spirit. According to an analysis of TCM's origins and development by Lin Shi from Beijing Normal University and Chenguang Zhang from Southwest Minzu University in China, traditional Chinese medicine is profoundly influenced by Chinese philosophy and religion. To date, modern science has been unable to explain the mechanisms behind TCM's effects.

The study is published online in Springer's journal *Pastoral Psychology*, in a special issue[2] dedicated to the psychology of religion in China.

The essence of TCM lies in its foundation in spirituality, religion, and philosophy, making it quite different from Western medicine and leading it to be viewed by some as magical and mysterious. Chinese medicine is an ancient discipline with a long developmental history and is very much influenced by religion and spirituality. Shi and Zhang's paper examines in detail six aspects of traditional Chinese medicine: its history; its fundamental beliefs; spirituality in traditional Chinese healing rituals; spirituality in the traditional Chinese pharmacy; spirituality in health maintenance theories; and spirituality of master doctors of traditional Chinese medicine.

This analysis shows, among other things, that the underlying premise of Chinese medicine is that the mind and body of a person are inseparable. To be in good health, a person must have good spirit and pay attention to cultivating their spirit. Chinese doctors see "people" not "diseases" and equate "curing diseases" with "curing people."

According to the authors: "Good health and longevity are what we pursue. More and more people are concerned about ways to prevent disease and strengthen their bodies, which is the emphasis of traditional Chinese medicine. It pays attention to physical pains, and at the same time is also concerned with spiritual suffering. Therefore, TCM can teach people to be indifferent towards having or not having, to exist with few desires and feel at ease, to keep the body healthy and the mind quiet, and to achieve harmony between the body and the mind and then to achieve harmony with the world and nature."

The special October/December 2012 issue of *Pastoral Psychology*, guest-edited by Al Dueck from Fuller Theological Seminary, School of Psychology, Pasadena,

CA, and Buxin Han from the Institute of Psychology, Beijing, brings together psychologists from China and the United States for an exploration of the psychology of religion. It discusses a wide range of topics on the psychology of religion in China including historical perspectives; religious traditions; religion, healing, and health; and spirituality and human development. This extensive special issue is a testament to the recent emergence and growth of psychology of religion as an academic field in China and to the growing dialogue between Chinese and Western academics and researchers in this field.

Do Palm Trees Hold the Key to Immortality?

Dec. 18, 2012 — For centuries, humans have been exploring, researching, and, in some cases, discovering how to stave off life-threatening diseases, increase life spans, and obtain immortality. Biologists, doctors, spiritual gurus, and even explorers have pursued these quests -- one of the most well-known examples being the legendary search by Ponce de León for the "Fountain of Youth." Yet the key to longevity may not lie in a miraculous essence of water, but rather in the structure and function of cells within a plant -- and not a special, mysterious, rare plant, but one that we may think of as being quite commonplace, even ordinary: the palm.

As an honors botany student at the University of Leeds, P. Barry Tomlinson wrote a prize-winning essay during his final year titled, "The Span of Life." Fifty years later, Tomlinson (now a Distinguished Professor at The Kampong Garden of the National Tropical Botanical Garden, Miami, FL) teamed up with graduate student Brett Huggett (Harvard University, MA) to write a review paper exploring the idea that palms may be the longest-lived tree, and whether this might be due to genetic underpinnings. Having retained his essay in his personal files, Tomlinson found that it provided an excellent literature background for working on the question of cell longevity in relation to palms. Together, Tomlinson and Huggett published their review in the December issue of the *American Journal of Botany*.

A component of an organism's life span that biologists have been particularly interested in is whether longevity is genetically determined and adaptive. For botanists, discovering genetic links to increasing crop production and the reproductive lifespan of plants, especially long-lived ones such as trees, would be invaluable.

In their paper, Tomlinson and Huggett emphasize that in many respects, an organisms' life span, or longevity, is determined by the period of time in which its cells remain functionally metabolically active. In this respect, plants and animals differ drastically, and it has to do with how they are organized -- plants are able to continually develop new organs and tissues, whereas animals have a fixed body plan and are not able to regenerate senescing organs. Thus, plants can potentially live longer than animals.

"The difference in potential cell longevity in plants versus animals is a significant point," states Tomlinson. "It is important to recognize that plants, which are so often neglected in modern biological research, can be informative of basic cell biological features in a way that impacts human concern at a fundamental level."

The authors focused their review on palm trees because palms have living cells that may be sustained throughout an individual palm's lifetime, and thus, they argue, may have some of the longest living cells in an organism. As a comparison, in most long-lived trees, or lignophytes, the main part, or trunk, of the tree is almost entirely composed of dead, woody, xylem tissues, and in a sense is essentially a supportive skeleton of the tree with only an inner ring of actively dividing cells. For example, the skeleton of *Pinus longaeva* may be up to 3000 years old, but the active living tissues can only live less than a century.

In contrast, the trunks of palms consist of cells that individually live for a long time, indeed for the entire life of an individual.

Which brings up the question of just how long can a palm tree live? The authors point out that palm age is difficult to determine, primarily because palms do not have secondary growth and therefore do not put down annual or seasonal growth rings that can easily be measured. However, age can be quite accurately assessed based on rate of leaf production and/or visible scars on the trunk from fallen leaves. Accordingly, the authors found that several species of palm have been estimated to live as long as 100 and even up to 740 years. The important connection here is that while the "skeleton" of the palm may not be as old as a pine, the individual cells in its trunk lived, or were metabolically active, as long as, or longer than those of the pine's.

Most plants, in addition to increasing in height as they age, also increase in girth, putting down secondary vascular tissue in layers both on the inner and outer sides of the cambium as they grow. However, palms do not have secondary growth, and there is no addition of secondary vascular tissue. Instead, stem tissues are laid down in a series of interconnected vascular bundles -- thus, not only is the base of the palm the oldest and the top the youngest, but these tissues from old to young, from base to top, must also remain active in order to provide support and transport water and nutrients throughout the tree. Indeed, the authors illustrate this by reviewing evidence of sustained primary growth in two types of palms, the coconut and the sago palm. These species represent the spectrum in tissue organization from one where cells are relatively uniform and provide both hydraulic and mechanical functions (the coconut) to one where these functions are sharply divided with the inner cells functioning mainly for transporting water and nutrients and the outer ones for mechanical support (the sago palm). This represents a progression in specialization of the vascular tissues.

Moreover, there is evidence of continued metabolic activity in several types of tissues present in the stems of palms, including vascular tissue, fibers, ground tissue, and starch storage. Since the vascular tissues in palms are nonrenewable, they must function indefinitely, and Tomlinson and Huggett point out that sieve tubes and their companion cells are remarkable examples of cell longevity as they maintain a long-distance transport function without replacement throughout the life of the stem, which could be for centuries.

Despite several unique characteristics of palms, including the ability to sustain metabolically active cells in the absence of secondary tissues, seemingly indefinitely, unlike conventional trees, in which metabolically active cells are relatively short-lived, the authors do not conclude that the extended life span of palms is genetically determined.

"We are not saying that palms have the secret of eternal youth, and indeed claim no special chemical features which allows cells in certain organisms to retain fully differentiated cells with an indefinite lifespan," states Tomlinson. "Rather, we emphasize the distinctive developmental features of palm stems compared with those in conventional trees." Tomlinson indicates that this reflects the neglect of the teaching of palm structure in modern biology courses. "This paper raises incompletely understood aspects of the structure and development of palms, emphasizing great diversity in these features," he concludes. "This approach needs elaborating in much greater detail, difficult though the subject is in terms of conventional approaches to plant anatomy."

Regular Jogging Shows Dramatic Increase in Life Expectancy

May 2, 2012 — Undertaking regular jogging increases the life expectancy of men by 6.2 years and women by 5.6 years, reveals the latest data from the Copenhagen City Heart study presented at the Euro PR event 2012 meeting. Reviewing the evidence of whether jogging is healthy or hazardous, Peter Schnohr told delegates that the study's most recent analysis (unpublished) shows that between one and two-and-a-half hours of jogging per week at a "slow or average" pace delivers optimum benefits for longevity.

The Euro PR event 2012 meeting, held 3 May to 5 May 2012, in Dublin, Ireland, was organised by the European Association for Cardiovascular Prevention and Rehabilitation (EACPR), a registered branch of the European Society of Cardiology (ESC).

"The results of our research allow us to definitively answer the question of whether jogging is good for your health," said Schnohr, who is chief cardiologist of the Copenhagen City Heart Study, speaking in the "Assessing prognosis: a glimpse of the future" symposium. "We can say with certainty that regular jogging increases longevity. The good news is that you don't actually need to do that much to reap the benefits."

The debate over jogging first kicked off in the 1970s when middle aged men took an interest in the past-time. "After a few men died while out on a run, various newspapers suggested that jogging might be too strenuous for ordinary middle aged people," recalled Schnohr.

The Copenhagen City Heart study, which started 1976, is a prospective cardiovascular population study of around 20,000 men and women aged between 20 to 93 years. The study, which made use of the Copenhagen Population Register, set out to increase knowledge about prevention of cardiovascular disease and stroke. Since then the study, which has resulted in publication of over 750 papers, has expanded to include other diseases such as heart failure, pulmonary diseases, allergy, epilepsy, dementia, sleep-apnea and genetics. The investigators have explored the associations for longevity with different forms of exercise and other factors. For the jogging sub study, the mortality of 1,116 male joggers and 762 female joggers was compared to the non joggers in the main study population. All participants were asked to answer questions about the amount of time they spent jogging each week, and to rate their own perceptions of pace (defined as slow, average, and fast). "With participants having such a wide age span we felt that a subjective scale of intensity was the most appropriate approach," explained Schnohr, who is based at Bispebjerg University Hospital, Copenhagen.

The first data was collected between 1976 to 1978, the second from 1981 to 1983, the third from 1991 to 1994, and the fourth from 2001 to 2003. For the analysis participants from all the different data collections were followed using a unique personal identification number in the Danish Central Person Register. "These numbers have been key to the success of the study since they've allowed us to trace participants wherever they go," said Schnohr. Results show that in the follow-up period involving a maximum of 35 years, 10,158 deaths were registered among the non-joggers and 122 deaths among the joggers. Analysis showed that risk of death was reduced by 44% for male joggers (age-adjusted hazard ratio 0.56) and 44% for female joggers (age-adjusted hazard ratio 0.56).

Furthermore the data showed jogging produced an age adjusted survival benefit of 6.2 years in men and 5.6 years in women. Further analysis exploring the amounts of exercise undertaken by joggers in the study has revealed a U-shaped curve for the relationship between the time spent exercising and mortality. The investigators found that between one hour and two and a half hours a week, undertaken over two to three sessions, delivered the optimum benefits, especially when performed at a slow or average pace. "The relationship appears much like alcohol intakes. Mortality is lower in people reporting moderate jogging, than in non-joggers or those undertaking extreme levels of exercise," said Schnohr.

The ideal pace can be achieved by striving to feel a little breathless. "You should aim to feel a little breathless, but not very breathless," he advised.

Jogging, said Schnohr, delivers multiple health benefits. It improves oxygen uptake, increases insulin sensitivity, improves lipid profiles (raising HDL and lowering triglycerides), lowers blood pressure, reduces platelet aggregation, increases fibrinolytic activity, improves cardiac function, bone density, immune function, reduces inflammation markers, prevents obesity, and improves psychological function. "The improved psychological wellbeing may be down to fact that people have more social interactions when they're out jogging," said Schnohr.

Exercise Can Extend Your Life by as Much as Five Years

Dec. 11, 2012 — Adults who include at least 150 minutes of physical activity in their routines each week live longer than those who don't, finds a new study in the *American Journal of Preventive Medicine*. Promoting the years of life that can be gained from moderate activity may be a better motivator to get Americans moving, said study author Ian Janssen, Ph.D., of Queen's University in Ontario, Canada.

Healthy Living Into Old Age Can Add Up to Six Years to Your Life: Keeping Physically Active Shows Strongest Association With Survival

Aug. 30, 2012 — Living a healthy lifestyle into old age can add five years to women's lives and six years to men's, finds a study from Sweden published on the *British Medical Journal* website.

The authors say this is the first study that directly provides information about differences in longevity according to several modifiable factors.

It is well known that lifestyle factors, like being overweight, smoking, and heavy drinking, predict death among elderly people. But is it uncertain whether these associations are applicable to people aged 75 years or more.

So a team of researchers based in Sweden measured the differences in survival among adults aged 75 and older based on modifiable factors such as lifestyle behaviors, leisure activities, and social networks.

The study involved just over 1,800 individuals who were followed for 18 years (1987-2005). Data on age, sex, occupation, education, lifestyle behaviors, social network and leisure activities were recorded.

During the follow-up period 92% of participants died. Half of the participants lived longer than 90 years. Survivors were more likely to be women, be highly educated, have healthy lifestyle behaviors, have a better social network, and participate in more leisure activities than non-survivors.

The results show that smokers died one year earlier than non-smokers. Former smokers had a similar pattern of survival to never smokers, suggesting that quitting smoking in middle age reduces the effect on mortality.

Of the leisure activities, physical activity was most strongly associated with survival. The average age at death of participants who regularly swam, walked or did gymnastics was two years greater than those who did not.

Overall, the average survival of people with a low risk profile (healthy lifestyle behaviors, participation in at least one leisure activity, and a rich or moderate social network) was 5.4 years longer than those with a high risk profile (unhealthy lifestyle behaviors, no participation in leisure activities, and a limited or poor social network).

Even among those aged 85 years or older and people with chronic conditions, the average age at death was four years higher for those with a low risk profile compared with those with a high risk profile.

In summary, the associations between leisure activity, not smoking, and increased survival still existed in those aged 75 years or more, with women's lives prolonged by five years and men's by six years, say the authors.

These associations, although attenuated, were still present among people aged 85 or more and in those with chronic conditions, they add.

"Our results suggest that encouraging favorable lifestyle behaviors even at advanced ages may enhance life expectancy, probably by reducing morbidity," they conclude.

More Evidence for Longevity Pathway

May 1, 2012 — New research reinforces the claim that resveratrol -- a compound found in plants and food groups, notably red wine -- prolongs lifespan and health-span by boosting the activity of mitochondria, the cell's energy supplier.

"The results were surprisingly clear," said David Sinclair, a professor of genetics at Harvard Medical School and the study's senior author. "Without the mitochondria-boosting gene SIRT1, resveratrol does not work."

The findings are to be published May 1 in the journal *Cell Metabolism*.

Over the last decade, Sinclair and colleagues including Leonard Guarente at Massachusetts Institute of Technology have published a body of research describing how resveratrol improves energy production and overall health in cells by activating a class of genes called sirtuins that are integral to mitochondrial function. The cell's power supplier, mitochondria are essential not just for longevity but for overall health.

Sinclair and colleagues had studied sirtuins in a variety of model organisms: yeast, worms, flies and mice. For the first three organisms they were able to thoroughly knock out SIRT1 and show that cells lacking the gene don't respond to resveratrol. But no one had been able to demonstrate the effect in mice, which die at birth without the SIRT1 gene.

In order to solve this obstacle, Nathan Price and Ana Gomes, graduate students in the Sinclair lab, spent three years engineering a new mouse model. These mice, seemingly normal in every way, were designed so that SIRT1 would systemically switch off when the mice were given the drug Tamoxifen.

"This is a drug inducible, whole body deletion of a gene," said Sinclair. "This is something that's rarely been done so efficiently. Moving forward, this mouse model will be valuable to many different labs for other areas of research."

The results were plain: when mice were given low doses of resveratrol after SIRT1 was disabled, the researchers found no discernable improvement in mitochondrial function. In contrast, the mice with normal SIRT1 function given resveratrol showed dramatic increases in energy.

While the tantalizing prospect of increasing healthy lifespan has made resveratrol the subject of intense scientific interest, some researchers have questioned the link to SIRT1. A competing theory holds that resveratrol may work by activating a separate energy pathway called AMPK, which, while also related to mitochondria, does not involve sirtuin genes.

In their new paper, Sinclair and colleagues report that when mice lacking SIRT1 were given low doses of resveratrol, AMPK was unaffected. When doses were significantly increased in these mice, AMPK was activated, but still no benefit to mitochondrial function resulted.

"Resveratrol is a dirty molecule, so when you give very, very high doses, many things could be happening," said Sinclair. "It's standard when you study molecules that you use the lowest dose that gives you an effect because of the risk of hitting other things if you use too much. But for the downstream benefits on energy, you still need SIRT1. Our paper shows that SIRT1 is front and center for any dose of resveratrol."

This research was funded by the National Institutes of Health and the Glenn Foundation for Medical Research.

On the Path to Age-Defying Therapies

Mar. 29, 2012 — One of the secrets to a longer, healthier life is simply to eat less. When subjected to calorie restriction (CR), typically defined as a 20-40% reduction in caloric intake with corresponding maintenance of proper nutrition, animals in labs not only live longer, but also have improved insulin sensitivity and glucose tolerance, both of which decline during aging.

Yet, for all of its benefits, CR's restricted diet is a stumbling block for most Americans. If only we had a drug that could do the same thing.

Well, we do, sort of. The drug rapamycin, which is used for immunosuppression in organ transplantations, mimics the longevity effects of CR and may tap into the same cellular pathway as CR. Unlike CR, however, rapamycin actually impairs glucose tolerance and insulin sensitivity, two hallmarks of diabetes. Clearly, rapamycin is doing something CR is not.

To understand better rapamycin's benefits and risks, researchers from the lab of Whitehead Institute Member David Sabatini and Joseph Baur, assistant professor of Physiology, at the University of Pennsylvania's Perelman School of Medicine, have discovered precisely how rapamycin is behaving at the cellular level. Their intriguing results are published this week in the journal *Science*. "We know that despite its adverse effects, rapamycin still prolongs lifespan, so there's a potential that we could make it better by just having lifespan affected and not induce the adverse effects," says Sabatini, who is a professor of biology at MIT and a Howard Hughes Medical Institute (HHMI) investigator. "The data in this paper suggest that it's possible."

Rapamycin, which is also called sirolimus and marketed in the United States as Rapamune, is a known inhibitor of the mechanistic target of rapamycin complex 1 (mTORC1), a protein complex that regulates many cellular processes linked to growth and differentiation. mTORC1 is part of a cellular signaling pathway, called mTOR, which responds to nutrients and growth factors. Mechanistic target of rapamycin complex 2 (mTORC2) is also part of the mTOR pathway and regulates insulin signaling.

Rapamycin has generally been thought to target primarily mTORC1. But work by Dudley Lamming and Lan Ye, co-authors of the *Science* paper and postdoctoral fellows in the Sabatini and Baur labs respectively, indicates that in mice, rapamycin also inhibits mTORC2, thereby reducing insulin sensitivity.

To see if rapamycin's positive effects on lifespan effects could be separated from its negative metabolic effects, Lamming and Ye bred mice whose mTORC1 activity was partially inhibited but whose mTORC2 activity remained largely intact. The females of this mouse population lived longer than control mice while maintaining normal insulin sensitivity.

"This shows that disrupting mTORC1 alone is capable of extending lifespan, if you can find a way do that," says Lamming.

For Baur, the experiments' results indicate that there is a possibility of identifying a better anti-aging drug than rapamycin.

"Our work highlights the potential utility of molecules that target mTORC1 specifically and suggests there is hope that by targeting this pathway, you could really get something that ameloriates age-related diseases without causing more problems than it solves," says Baur. "If you're taking an anti-aging drug as a preventive measure, you probably don't want to pay the price of diabetes."

How Calorie Restriction Influences Longevity: Protecting Cells from Damage Caused by Chronic Disease

Dec. 6, 2012 — Scientists at the Gladstone Institutes have identified a novel mechanism by which a type of low-carb, low-calorie diet -- called a "ketogenic diet" -- could delay the effects of aging. This fundamental discovery reveals how such a diet could slow the aging process and may one day allow scientists to better treat or prevent age-related diseases, including heart disease, Alzheimer's disease and many forms of cancer.

As the aging population continues to grow, age-related illnesses have become increasingly common. Already in the United States, nearly one in six people are over the age of 65. Heart disease continues to be the nation's number one killer, with cancer and Alzheimer's close behind. Such diseases place tremendous strain on patients, families and our healthcare system. But now, researchers in the laboratory of Gladstone Senior Investigator Eric Verdin, MD, have identified the role that a chemical compound in the human body plays in the aging process -- and which may be key to new therapies for treating or preventing a variety of age-related diseases.

In the latest issue of the journal *Science*, available online December 6, Dr. Verdin and his team examined the role of the compound β-hydroxybutyrate (βOHB), a so-called "ketone body" that is produced during a prolonged low-calorie or ketogenic diet. While ketone bodies such as βOHB can be toxic when present at very high concentrations in people with diseases such as Type I diabetes, Dr. Verdin and colleagues found that at lower concentrations, βOHB helps protect cells from "oxidative stress" -- which occurs as certain molecules build to toxic levels in the body and contributes to the aging process.

"Over the years, studies have found that restricting calories slows aging and increases longevity -- however the mechanism of this effect has remained elusive" Dr. Verdin said. Dr. Verdin, the paper's senior author, directs the Center for HIV & Aging at Gladstone and is also a professor at the University of California, San Francisco, with which Gladstone is affiliated. "Here, we find that βOHB -- the body's major source of energy during exercise or fasting -- blocks a class of enzymes that would otherwise promote oxidative stress, thus protecting cells from aging."

Oxidative stress occurs as cells use oxygen to produce energy, but this activity also releases other potentially toxic molecules, known as free radicals. As cells age, they become less effective in clearing these free radicals -- leading to cell damage, oxidative stress and the effects of aging.

However, Dr. Verdin and his team found that βOHB might actually help delay this process. In a series of laboratory experiments -- first in human cells in a dish and then in tissues taken from mice -- the team monitored the biochemical changes that occur when βOHB is administered during a chronic calorie-restricted diet. The researchers found that calorie restriction spurs βOHB production, which blocked the activity of a class of enzymes called histone deacetylases, or HDACs.

Normally HDACs keep a pair of genes, called Foxo3a and Mt2, switched off. But increased levels of βOHB block the HDACs from doing so, which by default activates the two genes. Once activated, these genes kick-start a process that helps cells resist oxidative stress. This discovery not only identifies a novel signaling role for βOHB, but it could also represent a way to slow the detrimental effects of aging in all cells of the body.

"This breakthrough also greatly advances our understanding of the underlying mechanism behind HDACs, which had already been known to be involved in aging and neurological disease," said Gladstone Investigator Katerina Akassoglou, PhD, an expert in neurological diseases and one of the paper's co-authors.

"The findings could be relevant for a wide range of neurological conditions, such as Alzheimer's, Parkinson's, autism and traumatic brain injury -- diseases that afflict millions and for which there are few treatment options."

"Identifying βOHB as a link between caloric restriction and protection from oxidative stress opens up a variety of new avenues to researchers for combating disease," said Tadahiro Shimazu, a Gladstone postdoctoral fellow and the paper's lead author. "In the future, we will continue to explore the role of βOHB -- especially how it affects the body's other organs, such as the heart or brain -- to confirm whether the compound's protective effects can be applied throughout the body."

Chapters from Physical Immortality: A History and How to Guide

Chapter 8: Your Spiritual, Energy, and Physical Bodies

One of the key concepts in this book is that you are not just your physical body.

These are concepts which are woven into many religions and philosophies, with related energy body concepts mostly being understood in the East more than the West.

Many believe that your entire being consists of at least three states as described below.

a.   The Spirit

Here we mean the spirit which is your "soul" or core of your being. An individual's spirit is one with the God spirit and is present in every person and every being. It exists outside of time and space. This is a place some call "no time and no space". It is everywhere present simultaneously.

The spirit exists in all things and each person has that same core spirit within them.

We can learn to live focused more in the spirit through a variety of religious, meditational, and philosophical traditions.

b.   The Energy Body

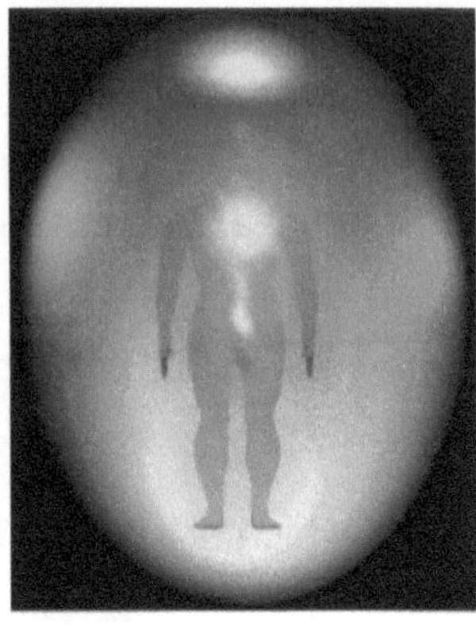

Figure 4-An artist's rendering of a Full Body

Some organizations like the Hindus and Theosophists believe we have multiple energy body levels. The Theosophists (9) believe there are at least six distinct energy bodies. Many other traditions only talk about one energy body which provides the life force to energize our physical bodies.

The acupuncture meridians and chakras are all parts of the energy body which exists in very close proximity to the physical body.

The aura is also a manifestation of the energy body too, which overlaps your physical body.

Many people claim to be able to see "auras" including this Author. The aura is the physical energy manifestation of the energy body. All living people have an aura and one can tell a lot about their health by how their aura looks.

c.   The Physical Body

This is the body most of us know, and that most of us think is all of us that exists. This is the body we want to heal and energize to achieve physical immortality.

Exercises done on the physical body also affect the energy body.

Herbal supplements work from the physical body to help correct energy flows in your energy body.

d.   How the Bodies Work Together

The concept of the spiritual development exercises, and physical exercises in this book is that they help increase the synchronization of these bodies.

By bringing the absolute peace and stillness of the spirit down into the energy and physical bodies you increase the perfection and health of those bodies.

This is since in the normal course of events the stresses of our life cause more randomness or entropy in our energy and physical bodies. These stresses of daily life age us prematurely and cause disease.

We can repair our energy and physical bodies by integrating them better with the spiritual body; and getting the energies to flow in the correct patterns, chakras, and meridians, and with more vital force.

The Spirit and Science Presentation

(Below is the text and slide numbers from a PowerPoint presentation in training course #7.)

1) About the Spirit: My beliefs are based on ancient teachings from Christian, Hindu and Buddhist beliefs. The concept is that we all having a core "spirit" which is part of the infinite and universal spirit.

2) The Spirit exists outside of time and space. Science acknowledges that before the "Big Bang" that created the universe that time and space did not exist. They were created when the universe was created

3) The Spirit exists outside of time and space. Black Holes are also an example of a place where time and space breakdown. All scientists can say is that in the center of a black hole, time stops and space shrinks to an infinitely small point

4) Quantum Physics and the Spirit There is a concept in Quantum Physics called "Quantum Teleportation" Quantum teleportation is the transmission and reconstruction over arbitrary distances of the state of a quantum system, an effect first suggested by Bennett et al in 1993 (Phys. Rev. Lett. 70:1895). The achievement of the effect depends on the phenomenon of entanglement, an essential feature of quantum mechanics.

5) Quantum Teleportation offers an explanation for how information can transfer over a distance with no time lag

6) Let's examine this phrase: Our health and vitality depends on how well these three bodies "Synchronize" together. Why is this?

• Because the spirit created the energy body and the energy body created the physical body.

• All three have "links" and the healthier these "links" the better one's overall health

7) Examples of bad synchronicity: Serious Diseases and Mental Depression. This situation may mean that a person's thoughts have created harmful thought forms in the Energy Body which affect the physical body to create the conditions for Cancer to thrive. Improving a person's connection to their spiritual core can also provide a stronger "life force" to their energy body which is then reflected into the physical body. (Ask Audience for examples) An Example of good synchronicity: Anti-Aging By living with a close connection to their spirit, an individual lets the high level of spiritual force enhance their energy body. This "High Frequency" life force then proceeds to "nourish" the physical body.

My own body: When I'm in a deep meditative state and I work to bring that state into my body, my physical body feels very calm, peaceful, strong, and healthy. I continually want my own body to feel like this.

8)   About the Spirit: Reviewing Previous statements:

That this spirit exists outside of time and space

This spirit is the basis for all of what we call "reality" or the physical universe

The spirit creates our energy body, which materializes our physical body

Our health and vitality depends on how well these three bodies "Synchronize" together

Long Lived Plants and Animals

Why Study Long Lived Plants and Animals?

- Because we have genetic similarities to them and therefore we can learn from them

- Seeing how they live in their environment can also give us clues about their longevity

- Some of these longevity records may inspire new longevity efforts for humanity

Clonal Colonies

- As with all long-lived plants and fungal species, no individual part of a clonal colony is for more than a very small fraction of the life of the entire clone.

- Some clonal colonies may be fully connected via their root systems—while most are not actually interconnected, but are genetically identical clones which populate an area through vegetative reproduction.

Individual Plant Specimens

- Many Plants and trees can survive for thousands of years—some in very harsh environments

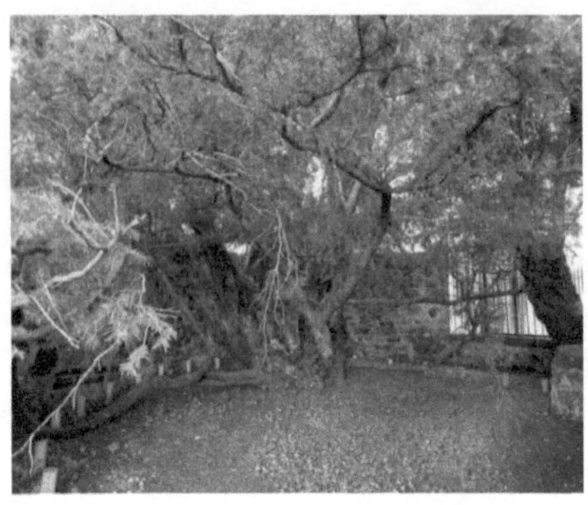

Fortingall Yew-Est 2000-5000 Years old

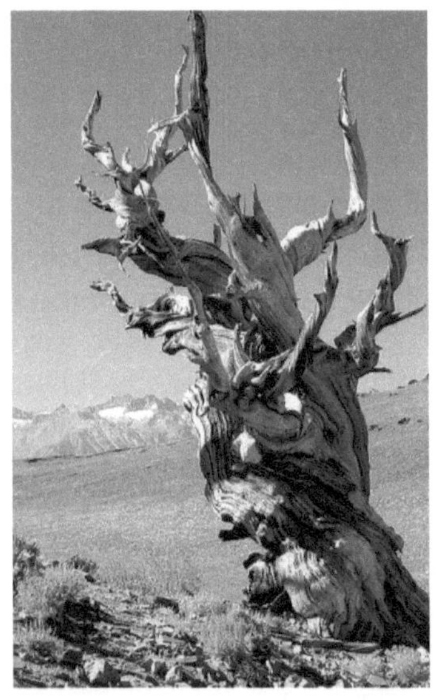

Methuselah-The World's Oldest Tree at 4,838 years old

Animal Longevity Records

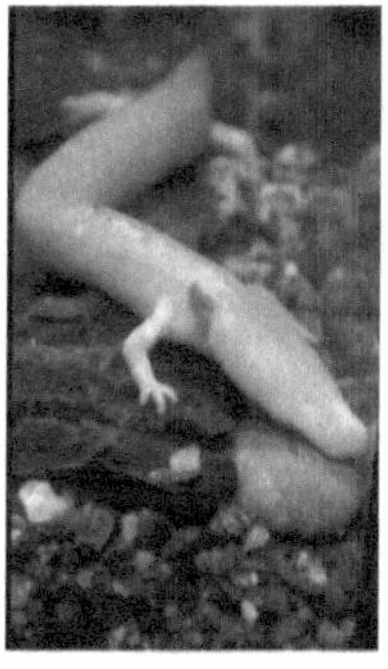

10. Warty Oreo- 140 years

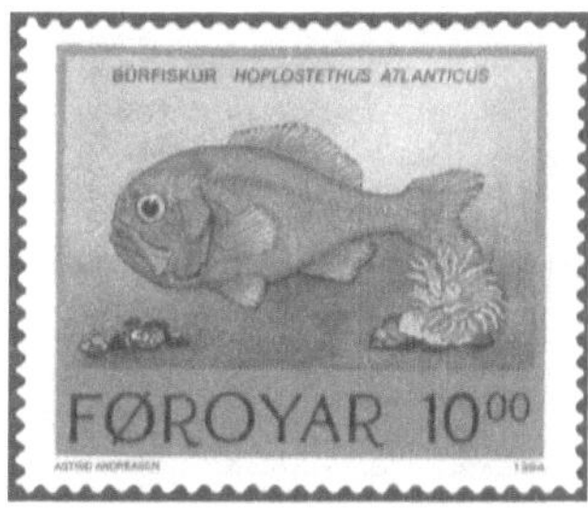

9. Orange Roughy-149 years

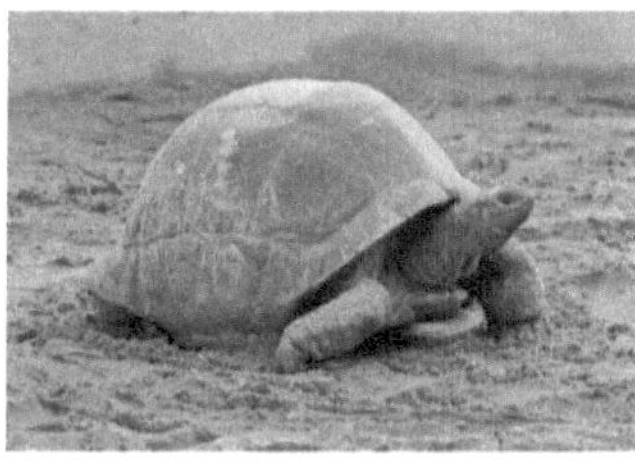

8. Aldabra Giant Tortoise-152 years

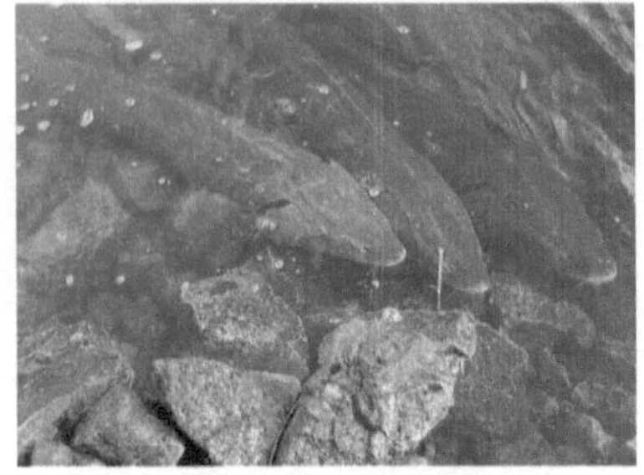

7. Lake Sturgeon-152 years

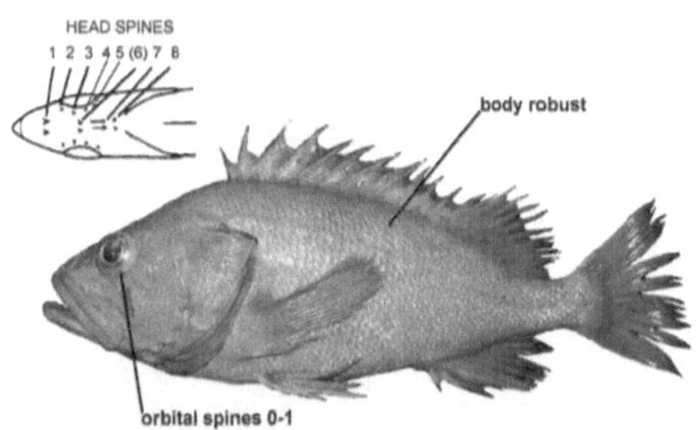

6. Shortraker Rockfish-157 years

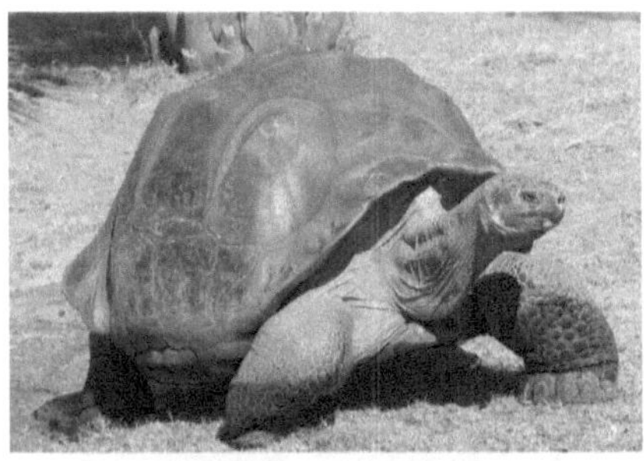

5. Galapagos Tortoise-177 years

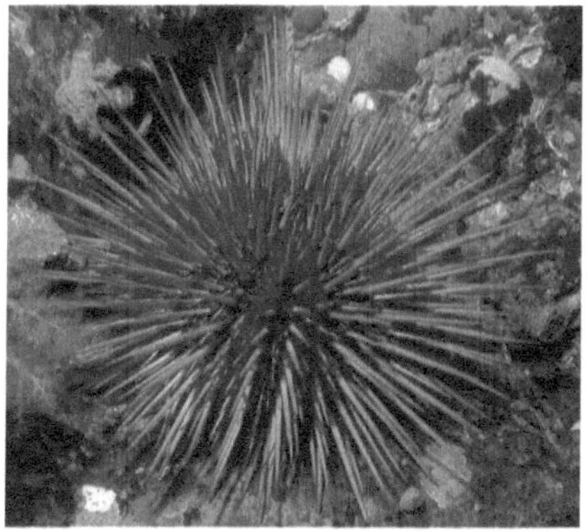

4. Red Sea Urchin-200 years (Kirt Onthank)

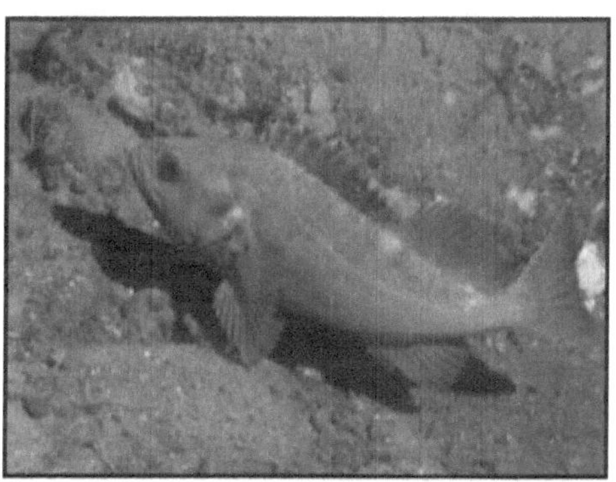

3. Rougheye Rockfish-205 years (National Marine Fisheries Service)

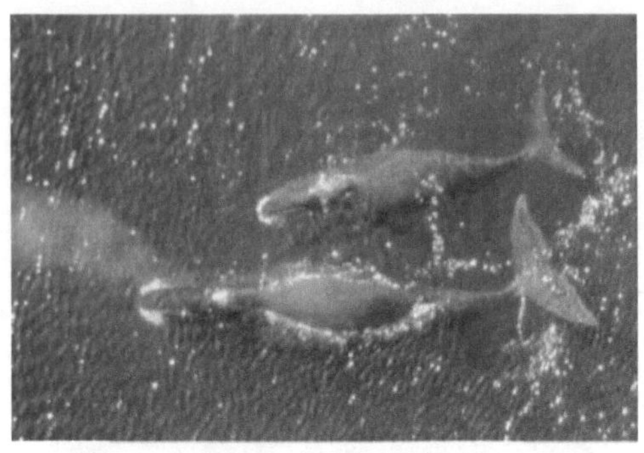

2. Bowhead Whale-211 years

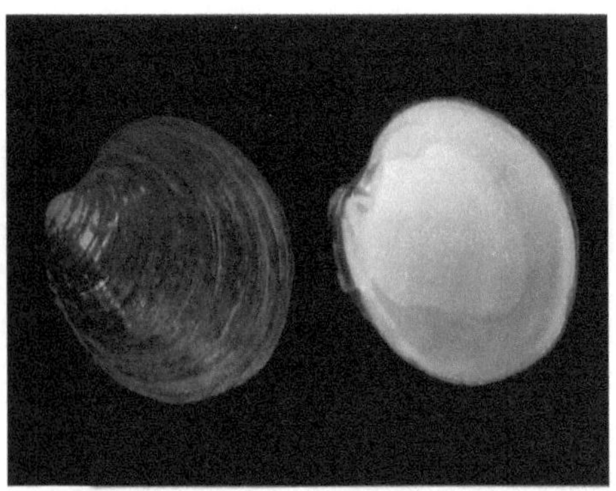

1. Ocean Quahog-400 years

Summary Questions

- Why do you think these animals live so long?

- What similarities do you see between any of these ten long lived creatures and ourselves?

- Is there something in their diet or environment which gives them such great lifespans?

Book-On Using the Scientific Method to Study the Paranormal

Chapter 4: THE SCIENTIFIC METHOD

a. What is the Scientific Method?

It is always a good idea to periodically evaluate one's progress personally in life, and in any field of endeavor. In science, we should also occasionally re-evaluate our models of objectivity to see how science is proceeding, and it may be that scientific objectivity overall needs to be re-examined.

Although many of the readers of this text may be well educated technically, I know that most technical schools don't specifically teach the history of the scientific method, so a review of the scientific method is called for to begin my case of how it should be updated.

This Scientific Method became informally popular during the Renaissance when scientists like Copernicus used his observation of the planets, and the fact that the earth was not the center of the cosmos, to show that existing theories of the cosmos were wrong.

Since then, the entire fabric of our civilization has been based on theory and experimentation.

Science is firmly based on hypothesis and theories, which can be objectively proven or disproven through repeatable experiments.

The history of the Scientific Method was also heavily impacted by three historical persons, who were also giants in philosophy, mathematics, and science in the last Millennium:

1) St. Thomas Aquinas

Saint Thomas Aquinas lived from 1225-1274 and was a Catholic priest who contributed greatly to the discussion going on at that time about Science Versus Religion.

A quote from a website on St. Thomas Aquinas [W4] sums up his effect upon western Christian faith and reason: Faith and Reason. -- The principles of St. Thomas on the relations between faith and reason were solemnly proclaimed in the Vatican Council The second, third, and fourth chapters of the Constitution "Dei Filius" read like pages taken from the works of the Angelic Doctor. First, reason alone is not sufficient to guide men: they need Revelation; we must carefully distinguish the truths known by reason from higher truths (mysteries) known by Revelation. Secondly, reason and Revelation, though distinct, are not opposed to each other. Thirdly, faith preserves reason from error; reason should do service in the cause of faith. Fourthly, this service is rendered in three ways: (a) reason should prepare the minds of men to receive the Faith by proving the truths which faith presupposes (praeambula fidei); (b) reason should explain and develop the truths of Faith and should propose them in scientific form; (c) reason should defend the truths revealed by Almighty God. This is a development of St. Augustine's famous saying (De Trin., XIV, c. i), that the right use of reason is "that by which the most wholesome faith is begotten . . . is nourished, defended, and made strong"

2) Rene Descartes

Rene Descartes [B7] lived from 1596-1650 and was known as one of the greatest philosophers of all time and was also the inventor of analytical geometry. His famous quote in Latin of "Cognito Ergo Sum" which translates to "I think therefore I am" was the result of a lot of his meditations on the nature of consciousness.

One of his most famous philosophical treatises on the scientific method is titled "Discourse on the Method of Rightly Conducting the Reason, and Seeking Truth in the Sciences", and it expounds on many aspects of consciousness including deciding what was truth and what wasn't.

In Part 6 of this treatise he remarks on the value of experimentation versus use of just the senses:

"I remarked, moreover, with respect to experiments, that they become always more necessary the more one is advanced in knowledge; for, at the commencement, it is better to make use only of what is spontaneously presented to our senses, and of which we cannot remain ignorant, provided we bestow on it any reflection, however slight, than to concern ourselves about more uncommon and recondite phenomena: the reason of which is, that the more uncommon often only mislead us so long as the causes of the more ordinary are still unknown; and the circumstances upon which they depend are almost always so special and minute as to be highly difficult to detect."

3) Sir Francis Bacon

Sir Francis Bacon [B8] who lived from 1521-1626 is largely credited as the father of the modern scientific method we use today.

A description of him by Voltaire (another famous French philosopher) credited Sir Francis Bacon as the person who made "experimental philosophy" a common feature of science in Europe.

A quote about Sir Bacon's work on experimental philosophy follows:

"In a word, no one before the Lord Bacon was acquainted with experimental philosophy, nor with the several physical experiments which have been made since his time. Scarce one of them but is hinted at in his work, and he himself had made several. He made a kind of pneumatic engine, by which he guessed the elasticity of the air. He approached, on all sides as it were, to the discovery of its weight, and had very near attained it, but sometime after Torricelli seized upon his truth. In a little time experimental philosophy began to be cultivated on a sudden in most parts of Europe. It was a hidden treasure which the Lord Bacon had some notion of, and which all the philosophers, encouraged by his promises, endeavored to dig up."
The civilization we live in today has been largely created by application of the scientific method, which was in large part formalized by the above three persons.

Our understanding of Science and Natural laws of reality allows engineers and others to create the things, which make our life easier. This includes everything from electricity to cars to spacecraft.

The Scientific Method can be expressed this way:
1) Develop a hypothesis of how something works
2) Make an experiment to test the hypothesis
3) Modify the Theory resulting from the hypothesis to conform to the results
4) Keep testing until the theory is proved or disproved.

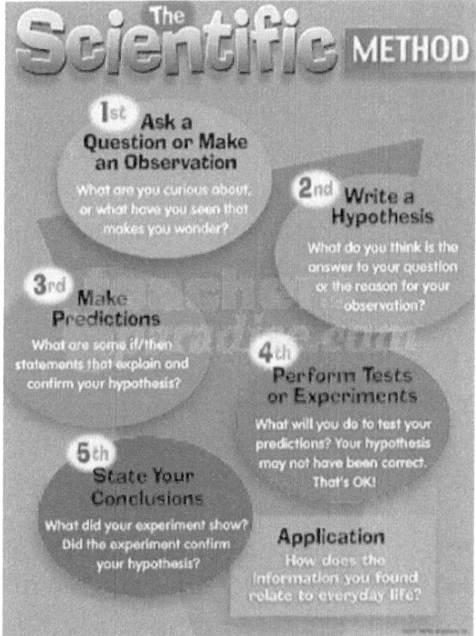

Figure 2-The Process of the Scientific Method

b. The Non Scientific Method of Observation

This has been the dominant way that man observed the world for most of his history.

Man would observe something then develop a theory about it.
There was no requirement that it was necessary to prove the theory to be correct or incorrect.

Thus some major misunderstandings about Reality were "Set in stone" such as the concept from Ptolemy in ancient Egypt, that the earth was the center of the cosmos. This flawed theory of the cosmos dominated for centuries and was probably responsible for holding back the true understanding in many areas of science.

Although the Roman Catholic Church has done many good works in history, it is also responsible for the stagnation of many areas of Science by holding church doctrine on the truth to be more important than real observations of the truth. In fact it wasn't until the 1990's—almost 500 years after the fact, that the Pope issued paper stating the Copernicus was correct after all.

Science versus Pseudoscience

It's critical to the understanding of my approach to a new philosophy to outline the differences between the scientific and pseudoscientific points of view.

Modern science is the foundation of our civilization and its methods need to be fully understood as well as its limitations to allow the reader to see where my thinking is proceeding.

Although in many parts of this book I criticize the Scientific Method , it has been critical to building the foundation of our civilization today.

Most people in the world have never been taught the Scientific Method so they don't questions events they observe the way they should.

Many of these non-Scientific Method people accept claims of events without the proper scientific scrutiny. This is a Pseudo-Scientific attitude which is too accepting of new phenomena and doesn't advance the scientific understanding of reality.

Most of human history has been written by people with this nonscientific attitude, and although civilization advanced slowly by trial and error,(such as the discovery of fire and farming); the lack of understanding of the fundamentals of nature and the lack of emphasis on repeating results limited advancement and caused false understandings of the ways things worked to continue for centuries.

Ignorance has led to many beliefs about God and reality for thousands of years which may have been wrong or incomplete.

One traditional example is the ancient's beliefs in the four fundamental parts of matter of Fire, Water, Earth, and Air. This sounds like a good division of matter, but has no underlying experimental observations to support these divisions.

Once people started really observing and recording Reality, they made progress.

The beginning of the use of repeatable observations was really the beginning of the scientific method.

The methods used to observe were primitive and depended mostly on the senses of the observer. Primitive could be effective though if the results were repeatable.

Many times though, people made a hypothesis based on their beliefs and didn't think it was necessary to test them for validity. This became pseudo-science and stunted advancement.

An example of Pseudo Science was that most people thought that life arose spontaneously from non-life until Evolution through Natural Selection became accepted through the work of Charles Darwin.

Subjective Versus Objective Knowledge

The scientific method is by its nature objective. In other words someone can independently verify all scientific observations with the right equipment and procedures.

This objective knowledge provides a strong foundation for building other science knowledge and technology, which makes our daily lives easier.

Subjective knowledge on the other hand is knowledge, which only the observer has. It has not been verified independently.

A good example of subjective knowledge is someone who has a strong vision of Jesus. The observer may feel that it was a real experience, but they usually can't prove it to someone through objective experimental results because only the observer was aware of the vision.

c. Can everything be measured objectively?

Today we have so much confidence in the results of technology from application of the scientific method that hard scientific advocates assume that everything can be measured by experiment and proven true or false.

The logical extension of this reasoning for most people is that if something can't be measured, it doesn't exist.

Now of course many people believe in God, and they know God can't be measured. Even many scientists profess belief in God.

This belief is not logical if God can't be measured. Right?

However, scientists also admit that there are many clearly physical phenomena which they can't measure either.

Examples might include:

1) What is going on at the center of the earth?
2) Are the fundamental constants of the Universe the same at a point several light years from us?
3) What happened to the Universe in the first instant of the Big Bang?

These are questions which may never be answered with objective scientific observation

This limitation is basically one of instrumentation. If you don't have an instrument to measure something you can't experiment on it to generate objective results.

An example would be that there was no way to measure radiation when the understanding of radiation was too limited to have already developed instruments to measure it.

This is an old problem which is part of what science is all about. Instruments have to be developed to make observations with the proper accuracy to prove or disprove a hypothesis.

There is a further problem with measurement:

Are there phenomena which exist in the world of consciousness which we don't haven't instruments to measure?

The anecdotal evidence is that the answer is yes—many people think they have experienced certain phenomena, (like telepathy) but we don't have any standard objective instruments to measure if it exists or not.

Here is another question to think about:

Are there events of consciousness which we can never develop traditional instruments for because they exist outside of our physical world?

The answer to this line of reasoning now becomes clearer—that there certainly are phenomena which we don't presently have the instruments today to properly measure. (How do you measure Love or Hate in a person?)

Even more discomforting than this is that there may be phenomena which we will never be able to measure even though we have a pretty good subjective idea that they may exist.

(How do you measure a ghost or a vision of the future—or the first instant of the Big Bang which created the Universe?)

We have become very confident late in the 20th Century that we are close to understanding reality and close to developing an integrated theory of all the physical forces.

We think we are close to final answers in the sciences and in shutting the door on ignorance and phenomena, which we can't verify objectively.

It's ironic that some scientists at the end of the 19th century also thought that they had discovered everything and there was nothing new to learn—just like the general feeling at the end of the 20th century.

Maybe the problem is that our vision of reality as proven by the scientific method is too narrow, and until we expand the scope of our thought to include a way of understanding other phenomena not so easily measured; we will never really get to a breakthrough understanding of reality.

We should also all have less hubris and more humility in our estimation of how far science has come and how far it has to go.

Chapter 6: TOWARDS A BETTER FRAMEWORK OF REALITY

a. Our Limited Understanding of Reality

Our scientific understanding of the world is only about 500 years old.

Mankind has existed for over 100,000 years, and the universe is billions of years old.

Is humanity so arrogant as to say that we have a close to final understanding of the natural scientific laws of the universe, or should we be more humble and admit that we only understand a tiny fraction of what is out there, and much more is undiscovered than discovered.

I spent many years reading articles and journals from organizations like the ASPR (American Society for Psychical Research) [W5] who have done good experimental work for 60 years on validating and understanding psychic phenomenon.

However if I were to go to the average person on the street they would say that these things have never been proven.

(I also read the standard scientific journals like Science and Scientific American.) Most scientists would also say that paranormal events haven't been proven to exist.

Instead of exploring how to understand and benefit from these abilities, most researchers in these areas are still being asked to prove that these things really exist. In this case many of the skeptics aren't really interested in the objective evidence because it would disrupt their cozy worlds.

b. The Scope of Reality

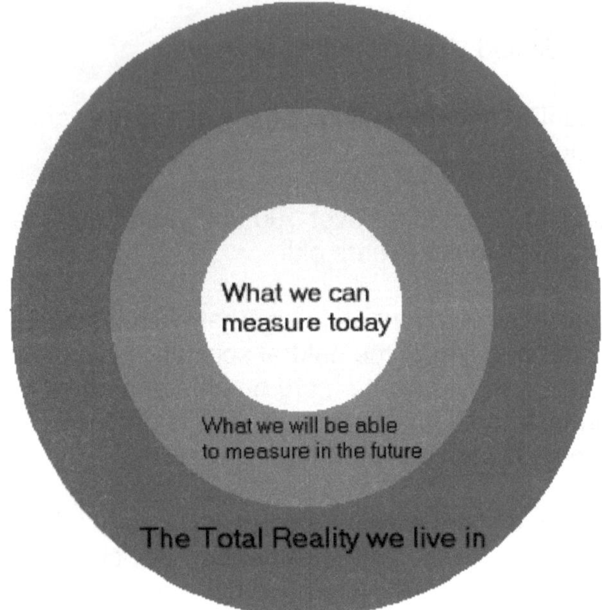

Figure 4-The Measurement of Reality

From the foregoing discussion on the scientific method and what is measurable, you can tell that I must have a significantly different idea of reality than the norm. Diagram #1 best illustrates my belief of our ability to understand Reality:

1) The inner yellow circle represents what we can measure with our instruments today and perform experiments on to prove or disprove theories.

2) The red circle is a larger area, which we will eventually be able to measure to understand and prove or disprove the way things are

3) The blue outer circle is the largest area, and is that part of the universe which we may be able to experience but will never be able to measure and validate with objective scientific approaches.

We may be able to subjectively perceive a lot of things in the blue area, but will never have the tools and techniques to objectively quantify it.

This blue realm may also include such things as where the soul goes after death, the fundamental nature of God, and certain dimensions of space and time, which we can postulate but never prove or disprove.

The red region may be more amenable to creative approaches for objective measurement and validation.

However, there will have to be agreement among the scientific community on some new approaches, which may constitute legitimate standards for objective measurement of phenomena.

This may include indirect evidence, which is used in areas like particle physics.

Neutrinos for example can't be directly perceived, but their existence can be inferred by collisions with other particles, which make cloud tracks which we can directly perceive.

The same approach should be transferable to validation of something like telepathy, where the medium of thought transference may not be understood at this point, but it can be validated through well-controlled blind studies and statistics.

I think that this type of validation issue of the objectivity of an experiment also presents barrier to further scientific progress.

Until new objectivity standards are set, we will never make good progress on a scientific understanding of consciousness and "nonphysical" phenomenon.

The Scale of Believability

When I was in my second year as an undergraduate engineering student, I had an opportunity to run a psychic research course during the 1975 January term at RPI under the auspices of the Chairman of the Physics department.
(He scheduled the course and I worked with him to develop the material and taught a lot of it.)

At that point I had also read a lot of books on metaphysics, and was a year into my own psychic development through meditation.

I was the daily instructor to a class of about 25 other students, where we did experiments on everything from pyramids to trying to hear messages from the dead on recording tapes.

In looking for a way to explain psychic phenomena to these students I came up with my scale of believability which I have become an ever-stronger adherent to as I've gotten older.

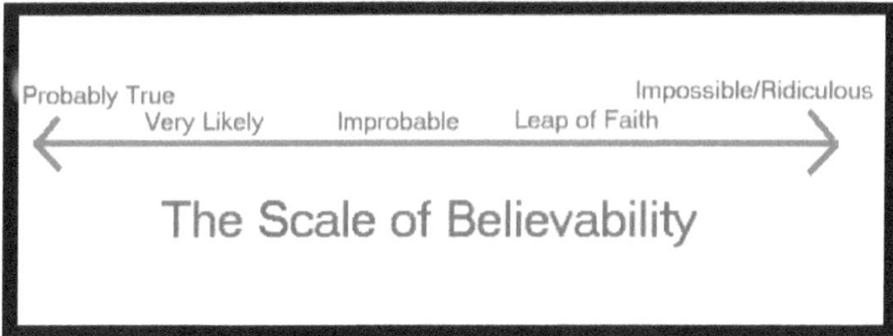

Figure 5-The Scale of Believability

The concept is simple:

Imagine a scale with one end called "Probably True", and the other end called "Impossible/Ridiculous"

Then start listing unusual types of phenomena along the scale as to where they fall.

An example scale might include the following key, with these sample entries:

Probably True
Very Likely
Improbable
Leap of Faith
Impossible/Ridiculous

Telepathy-Probably True

A very common occurrence is when you think of someone and they call on the phone right away; or how many married couples think the same thoughts at the same time.

Most people would agree because of these events, telepathy probably exists as a natural human ability in some form although it hasn't been validated by the accepted scientific standards yet

Psychic Healing-Very Likely

Many persons throughout history have reported natural healing from Christ to people in today's world. A lot of anecdotal evidence exists, and this is a common enough claim that most people would accept its existence, but they are still somewhat skeptical. Of course the scientific community doesn't validate this either.

Foretelling the Future-Improbable

Again, something commonly claimed. The standard story being someone who dreamed they saw a plane crash and then it happened. Now we are getting to something that is very subjective and can't be validated by today's scientific techniques.

Out of Body Experience-Leap of Faith

Many books are written on this subject, and thousands of cases have been reported, but it is a totally subjective experience and not measurable objectively today

Mental Teleportation-Impossible/Ridiculous

I'm talking about Star Trek beaming capability without the machines. This is really getting to the edge, but again if you search the literature, there are cases of this event reported throughout history although it is extremely rare.

Many more items can be added to this scale. I just wanted to use some sample ideas to explain the concept.

c. The "Real Reality"

After I made the preceding scale on Believability to organize some of the paranormal phenomena I had learned about, (and experienced some of) my next inclination was to try to create a dividing line as to what could be real and what was fantasy.

I found out I couldn't do it. Here is where I left the objective frame of reference and started to depend on subjective experiences, my logic, and my intuition:

I came to the pretty far out conclusion that not only does everything exist, but in the total of the "Real Reality" everything does occur, everything can happen, and everything probably has happened somewhere and sometime.

(The above statement has some similarities to the Buddhist and Hindu views of Reality which say that it is all an illusion. My statement also has some similarities to what science knows about matter which is that individual atoms take up very little space, and so the objects we see around us are really mostly empty space.)

In other words we live in a tiny self-restricted reality— anything you can think of is possible in some state, and ultimately there is no fantasy. Anything you can think of has some state of reality.

Does this mean the average person can think of a pink elephant and make it appear? It's Unlikely—but all things are possible given the right circumstances.

I know that this concept sounds insane, but it is the only view of reality which allows the explorer to think outside the

traditional reality box and set their own boundaries on what they can observe and do –not someone else's.
This concept is anathema to the scientific method because science is all about defining the differences between reality and what not reality is. If everything exists how can science determine what is really true?

Well, science has a wonderful purpose in giving us rules to let us mold reality, but most people get carried away into thinking that if it hasn't been proven it doesn't exist, which is a logical fallacy.

Can I prove my theory of Reality--No--but on the other hand many theories can never be fully objectively proven at all.

d. Fantasy and Reality are obviously different

There is an obvious flaw which most people would immediately perceive about my statements on their being no difference between fantasy and reality.

It is the simple observation that a cartoon dog on the television (fantasy) doesn't ever have the same physical impact as a real dog (physical) which you can pet and play with.

How can this obvious difference be rectified with the fact that are observations of these two things are different?

I propose that this difference is a merely a difference in the frequency and resonance levels of the two, and that the observer could tune into the cartoon reality through putting themselves in the correct state of consciousness.

e. On the Possible nature of Consciousness and Reality

One of my close friends and associates from my RPI days was Samuel Lentine, He was the blind Physics graduate student I've previously mentioned.

Sam went on to get his PHD in biophysics at RPI, and had at least three masters overall—in education, natural science, and physics as an educational basis for doing his experiments.

He became an instructor at RPI and did work in the BioPhysics department as well as starting a holistic clinic on the applications of psychic healing and psychotronics to everyday health.

Sam had a theory about the nature of Reality which ties in well to my own observations. I am summarizing his theory mainly from what I've listened to on taped lectures he gave during the 1980s to an organization called the US Psychotronics Association.

His theory was based on the idea of what he calls a "wave function" or "functional entity".

The basic premise of his theory was that all matter (and even space and time) has a wave form associated with it which is really a form of consciousness, and can be described as an extra dimensional attribute of matter.

You can call this energy the vital force, or orgone, or psychic energy, or consciousness, or many other names, but it is basically an energy field of the vital force of consciousness which is associated with every piece of reality down to the sub atomic level.

This belief is also in line with the Yogic and Buddhist religions which believe that all parts of the physical reality are conscious at some level.

Sam believed that this energy field contained an information imprint which described the nature and properties of every object, and that the physical object's properties would conform to the information which was imprinted on the energy field.

He also believed that this energy field could be described as a wave function and that it could be modified by other wave functions communicating with it and imprinting their waves onto the object's wave function.

One experiment he conducted was to imprint the wave function of the element radium onto water and measure the difference in the radiation count resulting. He claimed significant results from this experiment.

The experiment was done using psychotronic devices and mental manipulation to do the imprinting, and standard scientific instruments to measure and record the resulting radiation counts.

This type of experiment was performed using a hybrid of standard scientific instruments and psychic techniques which I have recommended as needed to expand the range of objective measurements needed to properly observe some of these phenomena under scientific conditions.

This theory would explain many of the paranormal phenomena which have been described, since many of them involve one object affecting another through paranormal means.

An example of how this works would be telepathy. Telepathy may work when the energy field or wave function of one individual communicates information which imprints the wave function of another individual. This imprint communicates the thought information to the second person which this other person understands.

How is this imprinting done? Sam and I both believe it done with some type of resonance between similar wave functions. Resonance occurs when two waves of similar frequency interfere with each other. The interference can enhance the target wave or cancel out the target wave depending on the amplitudes and structures of each wave function.

An example of resonance is the use of a tuning fork. The first tuning fork will cause the second tuning fork of the same design to vibrate when the first tuning fork is struck and the sounds waves transfer to the second one.

Sam's theory ties well into my own beliefs on Reality especially in what I describe as the "Scale of Believability".

If it is true that all physical reality is the result of the imprinting of information from conscious wave functions, then the idea that whatever a person believes can become reality makes sense.

This means that whatever a person thinks modifies the information content of their own personality wave function, and that the proper communication of this information to another person's wave function enables telepathy.

This also has impacts on the way physics, biology, and other sciences measure things because it means they are leaving out a significant component of reality from their measurements.

This view of Reality also does not contradict my views of God's relationship with man as Christianity propounds, it merely proposes a mechanism as to how this interaction occurs.

f. What is the Force of Will?

One more belief I have is in the power of a person's Will. What is Will Power? The dictionary defines it in part as-- used to express determination, insistence, persistence, or willfulness OR mental powers manifested as wishing, choosing, desiring, or intending

A person's Will seems to be a central component of their personality. This will also seems to be the driving force behind accomplishing anything in our Reality.

I think the human Will is also the driving force behind any of the phenomena discussed in this book.

People can develop their Will through exercise and experience like any other ability. (Have you ever noticed how two different people can say the same thing to a third person with different results. One reason for this is the will behind the person try to exert their influence.)

This Will can also be used to direct all of the actions both Psychic and non-Psychic which are possible.

Maybe one way of looking at Reality is that the individual's Will acts on others Will, and on the Will which created the Universe (God?) as a whole. (Is it blasphemous to say this? I don't think so, because even the Bible says that

God gave man free will, and man obviously can affect Reality which is God's overall creation. Therefore this is part of God's plan.)

The resulting Reality is a combination of the effect of all of these forces of Will.

We could also say that the Will is the uniquely identifying characteristic of a real Intelligence. Computers can analyze, but they don't have a Will.

On the other hand, even a worm has some type of will to decide what direction it bores holes in.

Will is the guiding influence which directs many forms of energy to accomplish or create things.

A person can therefore change the impact of themselves upon Reality by changing the force of their Will.

g. The Probability of the Future

One of the things I learned in my study of Reality was that everything has a probability of happening, and we can control those probabilities through our thoughts as well as our physical actions.

A physical action which could affect my future, would be where if I were to study in college and get a degree in Physics, I would increase the probability that I could become a PHD Physicist.

However, I'm not talking about just what can done through physical acts to affect one's own future. It is also possible to change the probability of an event happening through application of energy and information to the wave function for the probability event.

An example was one time when I was asked to join a football betting pool of about twenty teams and how they would do on the coming weekend. I didn't know anything about the teams, so I just mentally looked at the probability of which teams would be likely to win in a contest. I won the pool since my guesses were more correct than anyone else's guesses—even though the majority were very knowledgeable about the teams in question.

Another event which I've always questioned was my story about how I had a vision of getting hit by the surfboard, and then it later came true.

If I had made a real effort, I should have been able to avoid the getting on a surfboard in the first place and therefore avoiding the accident entirely.

Even religions like Christianity say that people have free will, and we are masters of our own fate.

I look at the future like we are in a river, going with the current (the time direction), and we have free will to navigate between the banks.

We also have an ability to look downstream and see rocks or shallow areas to avoid in the river. We can change direction to avoid problems depending on how well we look ahead, and take advice from our physical and nonphysical senses.

I had two other events which demonstrated to me the ability of a person to change their fate:

- When I was in the Renaissance center in Detroit in 1981, and had the mental warning of a mugging, I had time to stop and change direction before the attack occurred.

- I also had a warning of a possible disaster happening to me if I took a certain plane flight to Europe as I discussed in the chapter titled "Warning of a Disaster". I did not take the flight which crashed and am here to write this down as a result.

The probability of events occurring is another wonderful aspect of the Reality we live in.

Chapter 7: WHAT THE FUTURE CAN HOLD

a. The confrontation of Science and Spirituality

As previously discussed, there are two main camps of belief in Reality in the world today. These two groups I will call the "Scientific View", and the "Spiritual View".

Some people have feet in both camps, but most people belong entirely to one or the other.

There is a confrontation between the two groups, which can be characterized with the following imaginary points of view:

The Scientist's Orientation—

I believe in what can be proven by experimental evidence. Science has taken civilization out of the dark ages by grounding us firmly in Reality.

The spiritual forces like the Roman Catholic Church fought hard against early scientists like Copernicus who challenged the church's view of the way the heavens worked, and they were proven wrong.

If scientists hadn't challenged assumptions like these and others about reality, we would all still be living in primitive ways.

Religion and Spirituality are therefore dangers to scientific advancement, and people should be educated to the modern worldview, which has provided a standard of living unmatched at any time in the past.

I know from scientific evidence that what science can do to manipulate reality is real and true.

People who are ignorant tend to be spiritually oriented because they don't know anything better.

The Spiritual Orientation—

There are many questions people ask about who created us, and the purpose of life, which can't be answered by Science at all.

Science for all its wisdom doesn't have any better idea about the fundamental nature of consciousness that it did 100 years ago.

There are many experiences which people have had over the centuries, which can't be explained by Science; except to deny that the experiences ever happened. Is that really objective?

In fact, I know from personal experience and faith in my religion that it is real and true.

Scientists may have done a lot to improve our physical well-being, but is that an end in itself?

Is the ultimate aim of science for us to understand and control nature without any comprehension of the larger questions about God and our purpose on earth? This would not be a good way to live our lives.

a. A Simple Neutral Analysis:

* Both viewpoints have logic to them.

* Both views have good arguments that the other one could be a danger to our civilization if unchecked
* Both views seem to be diametrically opposed.

b. A Deeper Neutral Analysis:

The scientific viewpoint has only come into being in the last 500 years. Before that only the spiritual viewpoint had a real influence on the world.

Now that science is maturing, and is the driving force in the growth of civilization, it may have become arrogant in assuming that the traditional pure scientific view has an answer to everything.

Both views have elements of truth in them, but we are just at a point in our maturity as a race where we may be wise enough to integrate the best elements of both worldviews together.

c. A Synthesis of Science and Spirituality?

Some people feel comfortable with an integration of their scientific understanding of the world and their spiritual views or religion. St. Thomas Aquinas [B6] was one of the first great thinkers in history to work on a merging of the two, but most people still see them as opposing points of view.

How can we get the best merging of the objective information provided by Science, and the subjective information from the Spiritual point of view?

Here I would like the reader to see the benefits of such a collaboration:

What if people would realize that the quest for truth would only be strengthened by using both the Spiritual observations and Scientific methods?

Example #1—

Experiment:

A study could be done to measure the effects of spiritual healing on people using controls and procedures which most scientists could accept. The measurements should include both traditional scientific instruments and subjective evaluations from the patients.

Results:

If the results were positive and accepted, this would both expand the boundaries which science can explore to understand the energies of life, and provide evidence for more people to accept the benefits of that particular spiritual point of view

Example #2—

Summary

As you can see, science and medical research have lots to say about longevity and can give us some insight into things we can do to improve our own long term health.

This includes things like calorie restriction, resveratrol supplements, and relevant psychological attitudes.

That there are some entities which are virtually immortal. If we can learn how to apply that knowledge to ourselves we can live immensely longer.

Or even if we can learn to live longer like some animals and plants. There seems to be some genetic heritages which have much longer lives than others. With our abilities to change our DNA maybe those lessons can be ours too.

The future holds many exciting possibilities.

www.ingramcontent.com/pod-product-compliance
Lightning Source LLC
Chambersburg PA
CBHW031232250726
48655CB00005B/1911